Auscultation Skills
Breath & Heart Sounds

Fifth Edition

Auscultation Skills
Breath & Heart Sounds

Fifth Edition

Jessica Shank Coviello, DNP, APRN, ANP-BC

Associate Professor
Yale University School of Nursing
West Campus, West Haven, Connecticut

Wolters Kluwer | Lippincott Williams & Wilkins
Health

Philadelphia · Baltimore · New York · London
Buenos Aires · Hong Kong · Sydney · Tokyo

Senior Acquisitions Editor:
Shannon Magee

Product Manager:
Ashley Fischer

Production Product Manager:
Bridgett Dougherty

Manufacturing Manager:
Kathleen Brown

Marketing Manager:
Mark Wiragh

Design Coordinator:
Holly McLaughlin

Production Service:
S4Carlisle Publishing Services

Library of Congress Cataloging-in-Publication Data

Coviello, Jessica Shank, author.
  Auscultation skills : breath & heart sounds / Jessica Shank Coviello.—
    Fifth edition.
      p. ; cm.
  Preceded by Auscultation skills. 4th ed. c2010.
  Includes bibliographical references and index.
  ISBN 978-1-4511-8999-5 (alk. paper)
  I. Auscultation skills. Preceded by (work): II. Title.
  [DNLM: 1. Heart Auscultation—methods—Examination Questions.
      2. Heart Auscultation—methods—Handbooks. 3. Heart Sounds—
      physiology—Examination Questions. 4. Heart Sounds—physiology—
      Handbooks. 5. Respiratory Sounds—physiology—Examination
      Questions. 6. Respiratory Sounds—physiology—Handbooks. WF 39]
  RC76.3
  616.07'544—dc23

                                                          2013023781

Contents

Online audio cues

The following sounds can be heard on the companion Web site that accompanies this book.

AUDIO CUES

Heart sounds

Track	Sound
1	Normal S_1 and S_2 (base of heart)
2	S_1 (mitral area)
3	S_1 split
4	Abnormal S_1 split
5	S_2 (pulmonic area)
6	S_2 split during inspiration and expiration
7	Increased intensity of P_2
8	Increased intensity of A_2
9	Diminished A_2
10	S_2 split during inspiration and expiration
11	Paradoxical S_2 split heard during expiration
12	Persistent S_2 split
13	Persistent S_2 split in pulmonary hypertension
14	Wide, fixed S_2 split
15	Fused paradoxical S_2 split
16	S_3 over mitral area (S_1, S_2, S_3)
17	Abnormal S_3
18	Pericardial knock
19	Right-sided S_3
20	S_4 (S_4, S_1, S_2)
21	Summation gallop
22	Right-sided S_4
23	Opening snap of mitral valve
24	Pulmonic ejection sound
25	Aortic ejection sound
26	Midsystolic click
27	Innocent systolic ejection murmur
28	Supravalvular pulmonic stenosis murmur
29	Pulmonic valvular stenosis murmur
30	Subvalvular pulmonic stenosis murmur
31	Supravalvular aortic stenosis murmur
32	Aortic valvular stenosis murmur
33	Subvalvular aortic stenosis murmur
34	Tricuspid regurgitation (insufficiency) murmur
35	Holosystolic mitral regurgitation (insufficiency) murmur
36	Acute mitral regurgitation (insufficiency) murmur
37	Mitral valve prolapse murmur with click
38	Early diastolic aortic regurgitation murmur
39	Austin Flint murmur
40	Graham Steell murmur
41	Normal pressure pulmonic valve murmur
42	Mitral stenosis murmur (atrial fibrillation)
43	Mitral stenosis murmur (normal sinus rhythm)
44	Tricuspid stenosis murmur
45	Cervical venous hum murmur
46	Patent ductus arteriosus murmur
47	Aortic prosthetic valve sound and murmur
48	Mitral prosthetic valve sound and murmur
49	Pericardial friction rub
50	Mediastinal crunch

Breath sounds

Track	Sound
51	Tracheal and mainstem bronchi breath sounds
52	Normal breath sounds heard over other chest wall areas
53	Bronchovesicular breath sounds

Clinical contributors

SECTION 1   Heart sound fundamentals

Monica Narvaez Ramirez, MSN, RN
Assistant Professor
University of the Incarnate Word School of Nursing & Health
    Professions
San Antonio, Texas

SECTION 2   Normal heart sounds

Jessica Shank Coviello, DNP, APRN, ANP-BC
Associate Professor
Yale University School of Nursing
West Campus, West Haven, Connecticut

Helen C. Ballestas, PhD, RN, CRRN
Assistant Professor
Adelphi University, School of Nursing
Garden City, New York

SECTION 3   Abnormal heart sounds

Leigh Ann Trujillo, BSN, RN
Supervisor, Education Services
Education Services Franciscan St. James Health
Olympia Fields, Illinois

SECTION 4   Breath Sound Fundamentals

Mary M. Kelly, MSN, CRNP-C
Nurse Practitioner
Abington (Pa.) Pulmonary & Critical Care Assoc., Ltd.
Abington, Pennsylvania

SECTION 5   Normal Breath Sounds and
SECTION 6   Abnormal Breath Sounds

Shelba Durston, MSN, RN, CCRN
Nursing Instructor
San Joaquin Delta College
Stockton, California

SECTION 7   Other Abnormal Breath Sounds

Carolyn Spera Bruno, PhD, APRN, MSN, CNS, FNP-C
Assistant Professor of Nursing
Yale University School of Nursing
West Campus, West Haven, Connecticut

How to use this book

Auscultation Skills: Breath & Heart Sounds, Fifth Edition, and companion Web site with fully searchable text and audio cues have been designed to provide you with a practical tool to improve your ability to auscultate for these sounds and enhance your understanding of their physiology. By using this book together with the audio cues and referring to it time and time again, you can review each breath and heart sound until you recognize it perfectly.

This invaluable reference explains the physiology and pathophysiology of more than 40 different breath sounds and 50 different heart sounds. Illustrations highlight each system's anatomy as well as areas affected by—and auscultatory sites for—the sounds discussed.

The accompanying audio on the companion Web site provides electronically generated examples of nearly all the breath and heart sounds in the book. Breath sound examples begin with normal inspiration to make it easier for you to determine where the abnormality occurs in the respiratory cycle. Heart sounds start with the first heart sound to help you better recognize abnormalities in the cardiac cycle.

We recommend that you first go through the book and the audio cues sequentially, and then go through again to review the sounds that you find difficult. In the book, in bold type, a cue track number appears whenever you should play the audio to a particular track to hear a sound.

Use the pretests at the beginning of each chapter to check your understanding of the subject matter. If you are unsure of an answer, focus on that particular area of study as you read through the chapter. Then, after you have finished the chapter and listened to all accompanying audio examples, take the posttest to help you gauge your understanding of key concepts. You will find detailed posttest answers at the back of the book.

Throughout the text, you will find graphic icons that call your attention to important points. *Auscultation tips* advise you of sites and techniques to detect tricky sounds. *Alerts* warn you of life-threatening auscultation findings that demand an urgent response. *Age issue* is a feature that describes age-related differences in lung and heart anatomy and physiology as well as changes in auscultation findings across the life span.

For quick reference, we have compiled a glossary of commonly used terms and abbreviations and an easy-to-read chart of common disorders matched with their specific abnormal breath and heart sounds.

This edition also contains rapid-review flowcharts of seven common respiratory and cardiac findings that briefly describe what you're listening to, provide information to further direct your patient assessment, and detail appropriate diagnostic tests, treatments, and related care to give you a guidepost for further interventions. It also has a listing of English–Spanish phrases that you will want to consult when performing a respiratory or cardiac assessment on a patient who speaks Spanish. This resource will help you communicate more clearly with these patients and, thus, perform an accurate assessment.

The fifth edition of *Auscultation Skills: Breath & Heart Sounds* continues to be an invaluable reference for the young practitioner who needs to learn how to differentiate normal from abnormal sounds quickly and accurately. The text spans the simple to complex and acts as a wonderful review for even the most clinically expert in auscultative technique. This unique incorporation of didactic and Web-based audio simulation provides the needed tools for developing the skill of auscultation for today's clinician.

Why use this book?

THE JOURNEY TO A TRIED AND TRUE ART FORM...

The stethoscope was invented by the French doctor Rene Laennec, from Quimper, France. He believed that a more modern method to diagnose chest conditions was needed. To listen to his patients' heartbeats and breathing, he first used rolled-up paper tied with string and realized that the sounds were amplified in comparison to the ear directly on the chest method, which had been the previous practice. He struggled to find a name for his invention, discarding such names as "sonometer," "medical cornet,"and "pectrolique." Or "thoraciscope." Finally he chose "stethoscope," literally meaning "I look into the chest" in Greek.

We have come a long way from those early days but auscultation of the heart and lung remains a true art form. It is the end product of a marriage of the anatomy and physiology of the pulmonary and cardiovascular system with a practiced skill set. In this text, you will find that each chapter will provide the reader with a pretest and posttest challenge to the anatomy and physiology of underlying pulmonary or cardiac conditions coupled with posttest answers in order to help reinforce the information found in the text.

In addition, not only will the text generated by experts in the field provide you with the understanding of the sound generated from both heart and lung but the accompanying Web site will simulate the sounds associated with both normal and abnormal sounds. To reap the rewards of this time-honored method of evaluating the pulmonary and cardiovascular system, one needs to consider auscultation in the same light as a good consumer of music requiring a great deal of practice in order to train the ear. The editor requests that, in order to experience the full effect of this learning tool, you listen to the sounds heard on the Web site as you visualize the actual sound production in the heart or lung. This ties the physiology explained in this text to the sound generated and thus provides the reader/listener with a learning experience, generating a greater understanding of the power of the stethoscope.

In this age of imaging, auscultative skill has become an endangered species, the loss of which is a detriment to and enhances the cost of care for our patients. It is essential that the novice listener become skilled in this art form so that assessment skills can be applied in a multitude of practice settings where imaging may not be necessary, cost-effective, or readily available. For those of us who have provided care in underserved areas, this "on-the-road-skill" proves invaluable and is not dependent on the presence of technology. In addition, assessment expertise provides a day-to-day, hour-by-hour, and minute-to-minute evaluation in any fast-paced environment where a patient's condition can change rapidly.

We hope that you find this fifth edition living up to our previous standard of excellence of the past four editions and that this becomes a primary reference source for both learning and enhancing your auscultative skills.

Heart sound fundamentals

1 The heart and auscultation

PRETEST ▶▶▶

1. Where is the heart located in the chest, and what are the heart's dimensions in the average adult?
2. What are systole and diastole?
3. How do electrical impulses stimulate the heart muscle to contract?
4. Name the precordial sites recommended for auscultation of heart sounds.
5. Which sound frequency is transmitted best by (a) the bell of the stethoscope and (b) the diaphragm of the stethoscope?

ANATOMY AND PHYSIOLOGY

Heart location and size

The heart is a powerful organ. Its primary functions are to pump deoxygenated blood to the lungs, where carbon dioxide–oxygen (CO_2–O_2) exchange takes place, and to pump oxygenated blood throughout the body. The top, or superior, part of the heart is called the base; the inferior, lateral part of the heart is called the apex. The average-sized adult heart is about 4¾″ (12 cm) long from the base to the apex and about 3⅛″ (8 cm) wide at its widest point. The heart gradually increases in size from infancy through early adulthood, and usually is slightly larger in males than in females.

Right and left sides

Anatomically, the heart is divided into two functional sides: the right side and the left side, which are separated by the septum. Each side is further divided into chambers. The right atrium and right ventricle are the right-sided chambers; the left atrium and left ventricle, the left-sided chambers.

Each chamber has unidirectional valves that separate the chambers and control blood flow. The right atrioventricular (AV), or tricuspid, valve separates the right atrium and right ventricle; the left AV, or mitral, valve separates the left atrium and left ventricle. The semilunar pulmonic valve separates the right ventricle and pulmonary artery, and the semilunar aortic valve separates the left ventricle and aorta.

Dimensions of average-sized adult heart

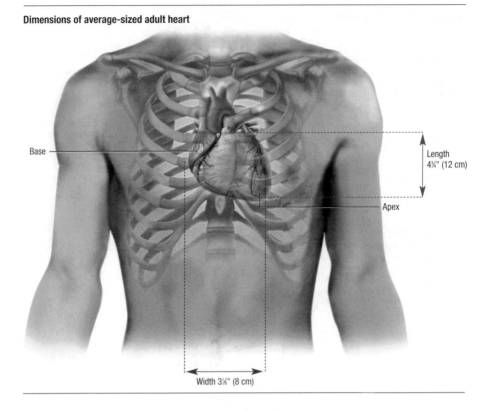

Base

Length
4¾" (12 cm)

Apex

Width 3⅛" (8 cm)

Blood flow

Deoxygenated, or venous, blood from nearly every tissue of the
body flows into the right atrium via the superior and inferior vena
cava. Venous blood from the heart tissue drains via the coronary
sinus directly into the right atrium. The deoxygenated blood collects there until the tricuspid valve opens, and then it flows into
the right ventricle. From the ventricle, it flows through the open
pulmonic valve into the pulmonary artery, which distributes the
deoxygenated blood to both lungs.

The complex process of CO_2–O_2 exchange occurs in the
alveoli. Then the oxygenated blood flows back to the heart via
the pulmonary veins and collects in the left atrium. From there
it flows through the opened mitral valve into the left ventricle.
When the aortic valve opens, the oxygenated blood flows into the
aorta, which transports it to all body tissues.

Internal structures of the heart

Superior vena cava

Branches of right pulmonary artery

Right atrium

Right pulmonary veins

Tricuspid valve

Chordae tendineae

Interventricular septum

Right ventricle

Papillary muscle

Inferior vena cava

Aortic arch

Branches of left pulmonary artery

Left atrium

Left pulmonary veins

Pulmonic valve
Aortic valve
Mitral valve

Left ventricle

Descending aorta

Systole

1. Aorta
2. Right atrium
3. Pulmonic valve
4. Right ventricle
5. Pulmonary artery
6. Left atrium
7. Aortic valve
8. Left ventricle

Heart as a pump

A healthy heart in a 154-lb (70-kg) adult pumps about 1⅝ gal (6 L) of blood per minute. Because the total blood volume in a healthy adult is about 1⅜ gal (5.2 L), the heart pumps the total blood volume of the body in less than a minute. It performs this task continuously throughout an individual's life.

An active process

The flow of deoxygenated and oxygenated blood through the heart, lungs, and rest of the body is an active process. The heart must generate enough pressure to pump blood through the arterial circulation. It does this by rhythmically contracting (systole) and relaxing (diastole).

During systole, heart muscle contraction raises the intracardiac pressures enough to systematically open the semilunar valves and pump a certain volume of blood. During diastole, the heart muscle relaxes, allowing the chambers to fill with blood again. This entire sequence is called the *cardiac cycle*.

Pathway of deoxygenated blood through right heart to lungs

Pathway of oxygenated blood from lungs through left heart

Deoxygenated blood

Oxygenated blood

The amount of blood pumped into the aorta each minute (cardiac output) depends largely on stroke volume. Stroke volume is the amount of blood pumped during each ventricular contraction.

AGE ISSUE *As a person without heart disease ages, his heart usually becomes slightly larger and loses its contractile strength and efficiency. By age 70, cardiac output at rest has usually diminished by 30% to 35%.*

Conduction system

Electrical impulses are primarily responsible for the rhythmic pumping action of the heart. These impulses are discharged automatically from specialized cardiac cells that stimulate the heart muscle to contract. The specialized cardiac cells and fibers within the conduction system work together to produce a contraction. The impulses fired from the sinoatrial (SA) node, located just below the entrance of the superior vena cava in the right atrium, normally initiate the cardiac cycle, and they usually travel along specific pathways.

After the impulse

When the electrical impulse leaves the SA node, it travels along the atrial conduction pathways located in the atrial walls, initiating atrial systole (or atrial contraction). The impulse rapidly reaches the AV node, located near the AV junction. From the AV node,

Diastole

1. Right atrium
2. Tricuspid valve
3. Right ventricle
4. Left atrium
5. Mitral valve
6. Left ventricle

Cardiac conduction

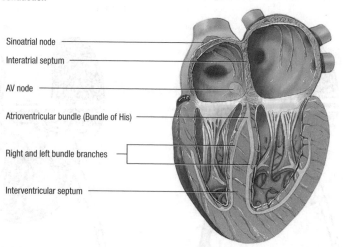

Sinoatrial node

Interatrial septum

AV node

Atrioventricular bundle (Bundle of His)

Right and left bundle branches

Interventricular septum

the impulse travels to the bundle of His located in the interventricular septum. Here, the bundle of His divides into the right and left bundle branches. These branches further divide into the tiny Purkinje fibers located throughout the ventricular walls. As the impulse travels through the bundle branches and Purkinje fibers, it initiates ventricular systole or ventricular contraction.

AGE ISSUE *As the myocardium of the aging heart becomes more irritable, extrasystoles may occur, along with sinus arrhythmias and bradycardias. In addition, increased fibrous tissue infiltrates the SA node and internodal tracts, possibly causing atrial fibrillation and flutter.*

Cardiac cycle

Several mechanical events occurring simultaneously during the cardiac cycle enable the heart to pump oxygenated blood throughout the body.

During atrial diastole, when the right atrium and left atrium are relaxed, blood flows into the atria. When the pressure in the atria exceeds the pressure in the ventricles, the tricuspid and mitral valves open, allowing blood to flow rapidly into the relaxed ventricles. The SA node, the pacemaker in a normally functioning heart, initiates an electrical impulse. The impulse is conducted via internodal pathways to both atria and results in atrial contraction. This contraction—atrial systole—pushes more blood from the atria to complete ventricular filling. The impulse is slowly conducted through the AV node, which allows time for the atria to contract completely and fill the ventricles with blood. From the

AV node, the impulse is rapidly conducted through the bundle of His and its branches. The Purkinje fibers receive the impulse and directly stimulate the ventricular myocardium. A forceful contraction of both ventricles opens the pulmonic and aortic valves and ejects blood into the pulmonary artery and aorta.

Unidirectional flow

The sequential and synchronized contraction (systole) and relaxation (diastole) of the atria and ventricles, along with the opening and closing of competent, properly functioning valves, ensure a unidirectional flow of blood through the heart and allow the heart to effectively move blood to all areas of the body quickly and repeatedly. However, this isn't a silent process. Auscultating heart sounds can clue you in to events in the cardiac cycle, such as the opening and closing of heart valves.

TRADITIONAL AUSCULTATORY AREAS

The heart's base normally lies beneath the sternum at the third intercostal space. Its apex is usually located between the fourth and sixth intercostal spaces, near or medial to the left midclavicular line. The apex is where apical pulses are taken and is usually the point of maximum impulse (PMI), the site where the heartbeat is seen or felt most strongly. However, to auscultate for heart sounds and murmurs, specific precordial sites are used. These sites are the aortic, pulmonic, tricuspid, and mitral areas and Erb's point. Each area is named after the heart valve primarily responsible for the sounds that are heard best in that location.

 AGE ISSUE *An infant's heart is positioned more horizontally in the chest cavity than an adult's heart. As a result, the apex is at the fourth left intercostal space and, until age 4, the apical impulse is to the left of the midclavicular line. By age 7, the heart is in the same position as the adult heart.*

 AGE ISSUE *In the elderly patient, degenerative bony prominences can shift cardiac anatomy downward or laterally.*

Locating the precordial sites

The aortic area is located at the second right intercostal space, close to the sternal border. This area is where the ascending aorta is closest to the thoracic cage and therefore where the sound of the aortic valve and the aorta are heard best.

The pulmonic area is located at the second left intercostal space, close to the sternal border. This area is where the sounds of the pulmonic valve and pulmonary artery are heard best.

The tricuspid area is located at the fifth left intercostal space, close to the sternal border. This area is where the sounds of the tricuspid valve and right ventricle are heard best.

Auscultatory areas

1. Aortic area
2. Pulmonic area
3. Erb's point
4. Tricuspid area (right ventricular area)
5. Mitral area (left ventricular area)

Alternative auscultatory areas

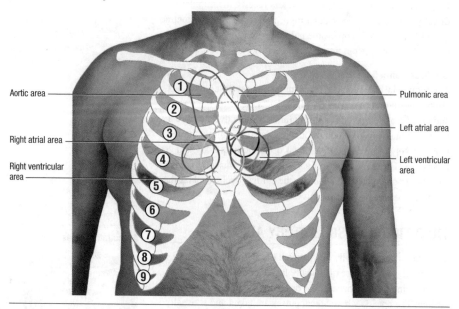

Aortic area

Right atrial area

Right ventricular area

① ② ③ ④ ⑤ ⑥ ⑦ ⑧ ⑨

Pulmonic area

Left atrial area

Left ventricular area

    The mitral area is located at or near the fifth intercostal space, just medial to the left midclavicular line. This area, directly over the left ventricle, is sometimes referred to as the apical area, or apex. The mitral area is where the sounds of the mitral valve and left ventricle are heard best.

    Erb's point differs from the four other areas in that it isn't named after a heart valve, but it's a good location to hear the sounds of aortic and pulmonic origin. This area is located at the third left intercostal space, close to the sternal border.

ALTERNATIVE AUSCULTATORY AREAS

Although the traditional areas are a good reference for auscultating heart sounds, it's important to know that the areas described can overlap extensively. Sounds that the heart valves produce can be heard throughout the precordium. Auscultation of heart sounds is not always necessarily over the anatomical site. Therefore, alternative auscultatory areas should also be considered when listening to the heart. (See *Alternative auscultatory areas*.)

Locating the alternative auscultatory areas

The left ventricular area is located from the second to the fifth intercostal spaces and extends from the left sternal border to the left midclavicular line. When the left ventricle is enlarged, this area extends in all directions. When the right ventricle is enlarged, this area is displaced to the left. The aortic component of the second heart sound, A_2, and a left ventricular S_3 and S_4 are heard here. Murmurs of mitral or aortic stenosis and mitral or aortic regurgitation, functional middiastolic rumble, and murmurs associated with hypertrophic obstructive cardiomyopathy (formerly known as *idiopathic hypertrophic subaortic stenosis*) are best heard here.

The right ventricular area is located from the second to the fifth intercostal spaces centered over the sternum. In severe right ventricular enlargement, this area may extend as far lateral as the PMI. A right ventricular S_3 or S_4 and the opening snap of the tricuspid valve are heard here. Murmurs of tricuspid stenosis or regurgitation and ventricular septal defect are also heard here.

The left atrial area is located from the second to the fourth intercostal spaces at the left sternal border. The murmur of mitral regurgitation is best heard here.

The right atrial area is located from the third to the fifth intercostal spaces at the right sternal border and may extend to or beyond the right midclavicular line in severe right atrial enlargement. This area is where the murmur of tricuspid regurgitation is heard best.

The aortic area is located from the right second intercostal space to the apex of the heart. The aortic ejection click and the aortic component of the second heart sound, A_2, are heard best in this area. Murmurs of aortic stenosis and regurgitation, increased aortic flow, dilation of the ascending aorta, and abnormalities of the carotid and subclavian arteries are also heard here.

The pulmonic area is located at the second and third intercostal spaces close to the left of the sternum, but it may be higher or lower. The pulmonary component of the second heart sound, P_2, and the pulmonary ejection sound are heard here as well as the murmurs of pulmonary stenosis and regurgitation, increased pulmonary flow, patent ductus arteriosus, and stenosis of the main branch of the pulmonary artery.

AUSCULTATORY TECHNIQUES

The stethoscope
The stethoscope allows you to hear heart vibrations that are transmitted to the chest wall. These vibrations have various characteristics: some are easily heard; others are less distinct. Consequently, the better the stethoscope, the better your chances of hearing subtle differences in the sounds.

Choose your stethoscope carefully. The chest piece should have a diaphragm and a bell. The diaphragm is designed to transmit high-pitched sounds more clearly, and the bell is designed to transmit low-pitched sounds more clearly. A flat, adult-sized diaphragm should be about 1⅜" (3.5 cm) in diameter and should be smooth, thin, and stiff enough to filter out low-frequency sounds.

Parts of the stethoscope

Headset
Ear tips
Binaurals (ear tubes)
Tension bar
Tubing
Bell
Stem
Diaphragm
Chestpiece

The bell should be about 1″ (2.5 cm) in diameter and deep enough so that it doesn't fill with tissue when placed on the chest wall. The tubing length can vary from 22″–27″ (55.9 to 68.6 cm), and its inside diameter should be ⅛″ (3 mm), or 1/16″ (5 mm) if the tubing is longer. The earpieces should fit inside the ears comfortably (covering the external ear canal), and the stethoscope shouldn't be too heavy because its weight can interfere with your ability to hear sounds accurately.

AGE ISSUE *Be sure to use the appropriate size stethoscope when auscultating the heart sounds of a pediatric patient. Most stethoscopes have an adapter to attach a smaller diaphragm. The bell is useful for pediatric and thin patients.*

Using the stethoscope

The way you use the stethoscope's diaphragm and bell affects the quality of the heart sounds and murmurs you hear during auscultation. To maximize the effectiveness of auscultation, you must hold the diaphragm and bell correctly.

To use the diaphragm, firmly grasp the metal area between the bell and the diaphragm with your finger and thumb, and press down firmly on the chest wall. If you exert too much pressure when listening with the bell, the stretched skin beneath it will act as a diaphragm, filtering out low-pitched sounds. To hold the bell correctly, grasp the diaphragm's outer edges with the index finger and thumb, and gently rest the bell on the chest wall. Look at the skin around the edges of the bell to see if too much pressure is being applied. If any signs of indentation appear on the skin, relax the downward pressure.

Also, remember to hold the chestpiece so that the tubing isn't touching the patient or you; such contact creates sounds that interfere with effective listening.

Auscultatory sequence

During auscultation, listen with the stethoscope over all five auscultatory areas, first with the diaphragm and then with the bell. Be sure to listen through several cardiac cycles to allow yourself enough time to become oriented to the sounds and to hear any subtle changes. Try to establish a pattern, and follow it methodically each time you perform auscultation.

Auscultatory sequence

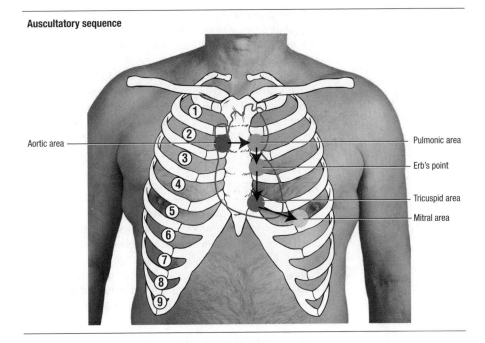

Aortic area

Pulmonic area

Erb's point

Tricuspid area

Mitral area

Performing the assessment
Before starting auscultation, place the patient in a supine position. You may elevate the head of the bed slightly if it's more comfortable for the patient. Then stand to the patient's right. Listen first with the diaphragm over the aortic area. Try to recognize the characteristic *lub-dub* sound of each cardiac cycle. After listening through several cycles, inch the diaphragm toward the pulmonic area. Try to move the diaphragm without losing track of the *lub-dub* sound. Then listen over the pulmonic area, Erb's point, and the tricuspid area. Continue in this manner until you reach the mitral area.

To locate the PMI, turn the patient slightly to the left, placing him in a partial left lateral recumbent position. This position brings the apex of the heart closer to the chest wall. Closely observe the chest wall for any sign of the heartbeat, which may appear as a rhythmic bulging. Then use your fingertip pads to palpate for the heartbeat between the fourth and the sixth intercostal spaces, near the left midclavicular line. The chest wall site where the heartbeat is seen and felt is the PMI. In a healthy adult, the PMI and the mitral area are usually located at the same site.

After listening over the PMI with the diaphragm of the stethoscope, turn the chest piece so that you can use the bell. Then, listen over the PMI with the bell. Reverse the auscultatory sequence, inching the bell over all the auscultatory areas.

If the patient can tolerate it, auscultate for heart sounds in supine, seated, and standing positions. Thus, after auscultating with both the bell and the diaphragm while the patient is in a supine position, have him sit up and lean forward slightly. Then repeat the entire auscultatory sequence with the diaphragm and the bell.

ENHANCEMENT TECHNIQUES

Ensuring the proper environment

A quiet, comfortable environment is recommended during auscultation for heart sounds. Privacy and a warm room are beneficial because the patient's entire chest is exposed throughout the examination. Shivering or any muscular movement interferes with heart sound transmission, making it difficult to accurately detect subtle characteristics of the sounds. Close the door and try to eliminate any noises in the room.

Some helpful maneuvers

Several maneuvers can enhance the heart sounds heard during auscultation. Besides position changes, you can also use maneuvers that increase or decrease blood flow through the heart. For example, you can have the patient squat or stand, hold his breath, or raise his legs while in a supine position. Another common technique is to have the patient cough several times or perform Valsalva maneuver. During this maneuver, the patient attempts to exhale forcefully against a closed glottis.

Another method that enhances the sounds heard during auscultation is to have the patient increase the depth of breathing. This decreases the respiratory rate and makes it easier to distinguish sounds originating in either the right or left side of the heart. For example, during inspiration, venous return is enhanced, accentuating right-sided cardiac events; during expiration, left-sided blood flow is enhanced, accentuating left-sided cardiac events.

You can help the patient by raising your hand slowly when you want him to inhale and then lowering your hand slowly when you want him to exhale. Caution the patient to breathe smoothly and continuously. If he holds his breath, he may produce a Valsalva-type maneuver, which will negate the cardiac responses being assessed.

◄◄◄POSTTEST

1. What is the heart's primary function?
2. How is the heart divided anatomically?
3. Name the four unidirectional valves.
4. What happens in the heart during systole and diastole?
5. What are stroke volume and cardiac output?
6. Describe the conduction of electrical impulses in the heart.
7. Briefly describe the heart's pumping action.
8. What are the names and locations of the five auscultatory areas used during auscultation for heart sounds?
9. Describe how to use the diaphragm and bell of the stethoscope correctly.
10. Describe the auscultatory sequence.

2 Heart sound dynamics

PRETEST ▶▶▶

1. How do heart sounds originate?
2. Name the two basic heart sounds and the valves associated with each.
3. How many characteristics are used to describe heart sounds?
4. How does the electrocardiogram (ECG) correlate with the heart's electrical activity?
5. How can you accurately document the heart sounds heard during auscultation?

HEART SOUND ORIGINS

The heart sounds heard through a stethoscope during auscultation are generated by vibrations from the heart's walls and valves and from turbulent blood flow. Normally, the heart's walls and valves are compliant as they move in response to pressure and volume changes during the cardiac cycle.

Blood flow

At the beginning of ventricular diastole, the ventricles are relaxed, and the aortic valve closes slightly before the pulmonic valve. For a brief time, both the atrioventricular (AV) and semilunar valves are closed. During this period, called *isovolumic relaxation*, intraventricular pressures continue to fall. However, the opening of the tricuspid and mitral valves follows quickly, and blood begins to flow passively from the atria into the ventricles. As the ventricles become distended, the rate of ventricular filling decreases. Then, as the atria contract (from stimulation of the atrial myocardium by an electrical impulse from the sinoatrial [SA] node), the ventricular volume is slightly boosted. The resulting increase in ventricular pressures causes the mitral and tricuspid valves to begin closing.

During atrial systole, the electrical impulse moves more slowly through the AV node and into the bundle of His. The impulse proceeds rapidly through the bundle branches and the Purkinje fibers, activating ventricular systole. Early in ventricular systole, intraventricular pressures increase above intra-atrial pressures, and the mitral and tricuspid valves close suddenly. Normally, the mitral valve closes slightly before the tricuspid valve.

For another brief period, both the AV and semilunar valves are closed. During this period, known as *isovolumic contraction*,

Valves producing first heart sound (S_1)

Tricuspid valve ———————————— Mitral valve

ventricular pressures increase, becoming higher than the pressures in the pulmonary artery and aorta. The aortic and pulmonic valves open, and blood is ejected through them. Normally, the aortic valve opens slightly before the pulmonic valve.

After a period of maximum ejection of blood from the ventricles, the ventricles begin to relax. As intraventricular pressures fall rapidly, a brief backflow of blood from the pulmonary artery and aorta toward the ventricles occurs. Reduced intraventricular pressures and the temporary backflow of blood are associated with the closure of the aortic and pulmonic valves at the end of systole.

BASIC HEART SOUNDS

A normally functioning heart produces two basic heart sounds: S_1 and S_2. (◆**Sound 1**) S_1, the first heart sound, is heard at the beginning of systole. It's associated with the closure of the mitral and tricuspid valves and the increasing pressures within the ventricles that cause the moving valve leaflets and cord structures to decelerate. S_1 is generated by the closing of AV valves and the vibrations associated with tensing of the chordae tendineae and the ventricular walls.

Valves producing second heart sound (S_2)

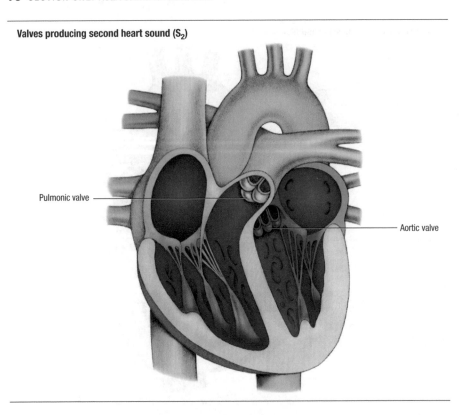

Pulmonic valve

Aortic valve

At the end of ventricular systole, ventricular pressures fall rapidly, causing a slight backflow of blood from the aorta and pulmonary artery. The decrease in ventricular pressures to a level below that of aortic and pulmonic systolic pressures and the temporary backflow of blood and recoil events are associated with the closure of the aortic and pulmonic valves. (See *Valves producing second heart sound [S_2]*.) The vibrations associated with these events produce the second heart sound, S_2, which marks the end of ventricular systole. (◆**Sound 2**)

Characteristics

Every heart sound has six different characteristics that need to be assessed during auscultation. These are *location, intensity, duration, pitch, quality*, and *timing*. If you keep these characteristics in mind each time you perform auscultation, you'll ensure a complete assessment of heart sounds, and you'll be able to provide the information necessary for an accurate and complete documentation. Also, because these terms are used universally, all health care professionals will be able to understand your auscultatory findings.

Location

A sound's location is the anatomic area on the patient's chest wall where the sound is heard best. Bony structures and landmarks, such as the right and left midclavicular lines, are used to describe the precise location. For example, you might document that S_1 was heard best over the mitral area.

Intensity

Intensity refers to the sound's loudness during auscultation. Usually, a sound's intensity is determined somewhat subjectively, based on experience. However, when abnormalities are present, intensity can be determined electronically by recording a phono-cardiogram (PCG) and by measuring the amplitude of the sound's vibrations. A PCG is a graphic representation of heart sounds that can be compared with the sounds heard during auscultation and with the heart's electrical activity recorded on the patient's ECG.

Keep in mind that heart sound intensity is related to the pressures generated and the blood flow velocity within the heart. It's also related to the patient's size, body build, and chest configuration. For example, a slender patient has a thinner chest wall; therefore, sounds are transmitted more easily through a slender patient's chest wall than through an obese patient's chest wall. Sounds can also be diminished by certain media, such as pericardial fluid or emphysematous lung tissue.

Duration

Sound duration refers to the length of time the sound is heard; it can be described as either short or long. Remember, heart sounds are brief vibrations that mark the beginning and end of systole. A sound's duration affects whether you hear it as a click, a snap, or a murmur. For example, murmurs are longer vibrations usually associated with blood flow during systole or diastole.

Pitch

The pitch of a sound is determined by the frequency of its vibrations. High-frequency sounds, like the notes of a piccolo, are best heard with the diaphragm of the stethoscope; low-frequency sounds, like the notes of a tuba, are best heard with the bell of the stethoscope.

Quality

Sound quality is determined by the combination of its frequencies. It may be described as sharp, dull, booming, snapping, blowing, harsh, or musical.

Timing

The timing of a sound refers to when it's heard during the cardiac cycle—that is, during systole or diastole.

The ECG

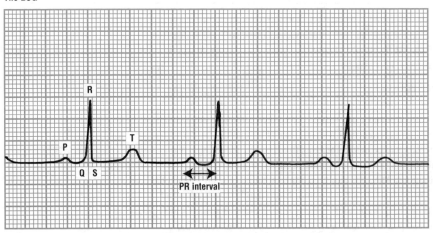

Putting them together

By using these six characteristics, you can describe precisely every heart sound, whether normal or abnormal. You can document what you hear, where you hear it, how you hear it, and when you hear it. Complete documentation also provides other health care professionals with invaluable information that helps them recognize subtle changes in the patient's heart sounds.

DEPOLARIZATION AND REPOLARIZATION

The sequential and rhythmic process of depolarization and repolarization is referred to as the heart's electrical activity. Electrical activity occurs at the cellular level in every contractile cell of the myocardium.

Initially, the contractile cell is polarized (in a resting state). Depolarization begins when the cell membrane becomes permeable to the flow of sodium ions into the cell. Repolarization begins when calcium ions move into the cell and potassium ions begin to move out of the cell. Then, the accumulated intracellular sodium and calcium ions are extruded while the lost potassium is restored to the cell by the sodium-potassium pump, completing repolarization. The cell is polarized to its original ionic state, and the myocardium relaxes.

The ECG

Heart sounds are produced by mechanical events that occur in response to an electrical impulse originating in the SA node. This electrical impulse travels through the myocardium, activating the atria and ventricles. The ECG documents the timing and

Graphically documenting S₁ and S₂

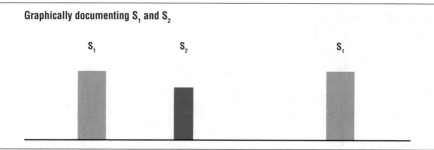

amplitude of the heart's electrical activity but doesn't reflect the mechanical events in the heart.

The ECG correlates with the heart's electrical activity in the following manner. The SA node fires, and the impulse spreads through the atria. The P wave, which is part of the ECG waveform, represents atrial depolarization. Atrial contraction is stimulated by and closely follows atrial depolarization. The QRS complex represents electrical depolarization of the ventricles. Atrial repolarization isn't seen in the ECG because it's hidden in the PR segment and the QRS complex. The T wave represents ventricular repolarization.

The impulse travels through the AV node, the bundle of His, the bundle branches, and the Purkinje fibers before the ventricles contract. The time between atrial depolarization and ventricular depolarization is recorded in the ECG as the PR interval: it begins at the onset of the P wave and lasts until the onset of the QRS complex. The time interval of the PR interval correlates with the time interval between atrial contraction and ventricular contraction.

ECG's relationship to first and second heart sounds

The first and second heart sounds directly correlate with a patient's ECG. S_1 normally occurs just after the QRS complex; S_2, at the end of the T wave. (See *Correlation of S_1 and S_2 with ECG*, page 20.)

DOCUMENTING HEART SOUNDS

The characteristics of each heart sound must be thoroughly documented. A PCG provides one method of graphically representing heart sounds. (See *PCG and ECG showing S_1 and S_2*, page 20.) However, it isn't used routinely for every patient; therefore, a more practical graphic method of documenting heart sounds is recommended.

The intensity, duration, and timing of heart sounds can be represented graphically as rectangular blocks placed perpendicularly on a horizontal baseline. The block's height corresponds to

Correlation of S₁ and S₂ with ECG

PCG and ECG showing S₁ and S₂

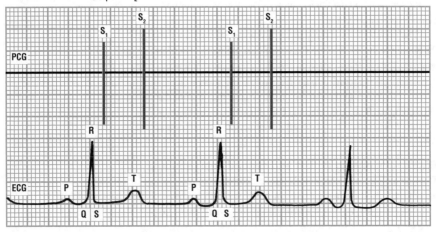

the heart sound's intensity (the higher the intensity, the higher the block); the block's width, to the duration of the sound.

The proximity of one block on the baseline to the next block represents the time interval between one sound and another. The spacing between the blocks can also be used to specify the relationship of a particular heart sound to systole or diastole.

◀◀◀POSTTEST

1. How is S_1 generated?
2. How is S_2 generated?
3. What is a heart sound's location?
4. What is a heart sound's intensity?
5. What is a heart sound's duration?
6. What is a heart sound's pitch?
7. What is a heart sound's quality?
8. What is a heart sound's timing?
9. Describe how the ECG correlates with the heart's electrical activity.
10. When do S_1 and S_2 occur in relation to the ECG waveform?

2

Normal heart sounds

The first heart sound

PRETEST ◆◆◆

1. What produces the first heart sound (S_1)?
2. What are the two basic components of S_1?
3. Where is S_1 heard best?
4. Describe S_1, using six characteristics.
5. What is a widened S_1 split?

Valves involved in S_1 sound production

1. Mitral valve
2. Tricuspid valve

Auscultatory area for S_1

Mitral area

NORMAL S_1

The cardiac vibrations associated with the closure of the mitral and tricuspid valves produce the first heart sound, S_1. (◆Sound 2) Normally, only two components of the first heart sound are audible. The first component, referred to as M_1, is associated with the closure of the mitral valve; the second component, T_1, is associated with the closure of the tricuspid valve. Both valves close at the beginning of ventricular systole, but the mitral valve usually closes slightly ahead of the tricuspid valve.

Auscultatory area and relationship to ECG

M_1 and T_1 are usually perceived as a single sound called S_1, which is heard best near the apex of the heart over the mitral area, using the diaphragm of the stethoscope. A single sound is heard because left-sided heart sounds are normally more intense at this site. S_1 occurs just after the QRS complex on the electrocardiogram (ECG) waveform.

As you inch the stethoscope from the mitral area toward the tricuspid area, without losing track of S_1, the M_1 and T_1 components of S_1 may become evident. Expiration makes them easier to hear. (◆Sound 3) T_1 trails M_1 slightly and is softer; it's heard best near the left sternal border. The timing of M_1 and T_1 with the QRS complex remains the same. In many patients, only the first heart sound is heard because M_1 and T_1 are separated by a 20-millisecond—or shorter—pause, which the human ear perceives as one sound. (See *PCG and ECG showing normal S_1 split*, page 26.)

AUSCULTATION TIP *If S_1 is difficult to identify, palpate for the carotid pulse while performing auscultation. S_1 will occur just before you feel the carotid pulse.*

PCG and ECG showing S₁

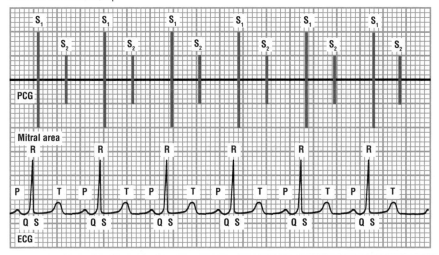

Sound characteristics

S_1 is usually heard best near the heart's apex over the mitral area. Its intensity directly relates to the force of ventricular contraction and the ECG PR interval. The shorter the PR interval, the more widely open the mitral and tricuspid leaflets are at the onset of ventricular contraction. Thus, the distance they must be moved is greater, causing more intense vibrations when they close and a louder S_1. S_1 is short in duration. You can hear its high pitch best with the diaphragm of the stethoscope. The quality of S_1 is somewhat dull. The S_1 timing coincides with the beginning of ventricular systole and just precedes a palpable carotid pulse. (◆**Sound 2**) The characteristics of the normally split S_1 into M_1 and T_1 are the same. (◆**Sound 3**)

Enhancing S₁

S_1 can be enhanced by sympathetic stimulation, such as that provided by a brief period of exercise.

Auscultatory area for M₁ and T₁

1. Tricuspid area
2. Mitral area

PCG and ECG showing normal S₁ split

PCG and ECG showing abnormal S₁ split

ABNORMAL S₁ SPLIT

Widened S₁ split

The normal M_1-T_1 split heard over the tricuspid area widens when electrical activation and contraction of the right ventricle are delayed. Such a delay causes delayed tricuspid valve closure. (◆**Sound 4**) This abnormal finding is associated with complete right bundle branch block, left ventricular ectopic beats, epicardial pacing of the left ventricle, tricuspid stenosis, atrial septal defect, Ebstein's anomaly, and left ventricular tachycardia.

Auscultatory area for abnormal S₁ split

Tricuspid area ——

◀◀◀POSTTEST

1. What produces S_1?
2. What are the components of S_1?
3. Where is S_1 heard best during auscultation, and how does it change as the stethoscope is inched from one area to another?
4. Describe the characteristics of S_1.
5. How can S_1 be enhanced?
6. When does an abnormal S_1 split occur?
7. Which conditions are associated with an abnormal S_1 split?

4 The second heart sound

PRETEST ◆◆◆

1. How does the second heart sound (S_2) differ from the first heart sound (S_1)?
2. What are the components of S_2?
3. Describe the characteristics of S_2.
4. What is an S_2 split?
5. Which types of S_2 splits may be heard during auscultation?

Valves involved in S_2 sound production

1. Aortic valve
2. Pulmonic valve

NORMAL S_2

The cardiac vibrations associated with the closure of the aortic and pulmonic valves produce the second heart sound, S_2. S_2 is usually louder than S_1 at the heart's base and usually slightly higher in pitch than S_1 at the heart's apex.

S_2, like S_1, has two basic components: the aortic (A_2) component and the pulmonic (P_2) component. Both valves close at the end of ventricular systole. Normally, the aortic valve closes slightly ahead of the pulmonic valve.

The closing pressure is higher in the aorta than in the pulmonary artery; therefore, A_2 usually occurs earlier and is louder than P_2. (◆**Sound 5**) Furthermore, A_2 can be heard over the entire precordium, whereas P_2 is usually auscultated over the pulmonic area.

Auscultatory area and relationship to ECG

To hear both components of S_2, listen carefully with the diaphragm of the stethoscope over the pulmonic area. Listen for S_2 just after the T wave in the patient's electrocardiogram (ECG).

Sound characteristics

S_2 is usually heard best near the heart's base, over the pulmonic area or over Erb's point. Its intensity directly relates to the amount of closing pressure in the aorta and pulmonary artery. S_2 is slightly shorter in duration than S_1. You can hear its high pitch best with the diaphragm of the stethoscope. The quality of S_2 is somewhat booming; its timing coincides with the end of ventricular systole. (◆**Sound 5**)

PCG and ECG showing S₂

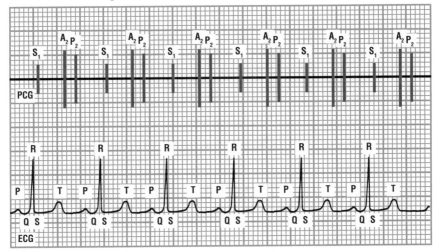

S₂ SPLIT SOUNDS

Normal S₂ split

The splitting of S₂ into the A₂ and P₂ components is heard best during inspiration over Erb's point.

> **AGE ISSUE** *Normal splitting of S₂ in children may be heard in the second left intercostal space. The splitting of S₂ in elderly persons may be more difficult to hear because of the widening of the anteroposterior chest diameter.*

Remember, inspiration causes an increase in the venous return to the right side of the heart. This increased venous return prolongs the right ventricular ejection time. Inspiration also reduces pressure in the pulmonary artery, resulting in a delayed P₂ or closure of the pulmonic valve. A decrease in blood flow to the left side of the heart occurs simultaneously, resulting in a shorter left ventricular ejection time.

Therefore, A₂ is heard earlier than P₂. (◆**Sound 6**) This means that a normal S₂ split is heard during inspiration, and the A₂ and P₂ components fuse during expiration.

Auscultatory area for S₂

1. Pulmonic area
2. Erb's point

Auscultatory area for normal S₂ split

Erb's point

PCG and ECG showing respiratory changes in normal S₂ split

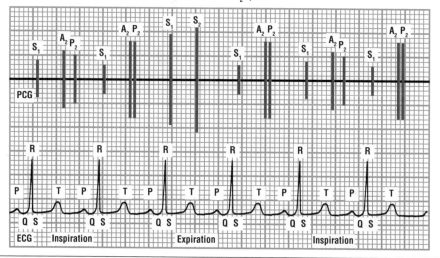

While listening to S_2, you must determine the intensity of the A_2 and P_2 components and note the duration of the A_2-P_2 interval as well as its relationship to the respiratory cycle. (**◆Sound 6**) You should also document the S_2 split, noting whether the A_2-P_2 interval increases or decreases during inspiration and expiration.

Changes in A₂ and P₂ intensity

The intensity of A_2 and P_2 changes proportionally with the difference in pressure gradients across the closed aortic and pulmonic valves. For example, P_2 may be louder than normal in conditions associated with elevated pulmonary artery diastolic pressure, as occurs in some patients with heart failure, mitral stenosis, Eisenmenger's syndrome, or other congenital heart diseases. When P_2 increases in intensity, it's sometimes heard over the mitral area and along the left sternal border. (**◆Sound 7**)

A_2 intensity increases when diastolic pressure in the aorta increases. (**◆Sound 8**) This commonly happens during exercise; during states of excitement such as extreme fear; in hyperkinetic conditions, such as thyrotoxicosis, fever, and pregnancy; and in systemic hypertension. However, if the patient has left ventricular decompensation, ventricular relaxation is slower, and the pressure gradients may not be great enough to produce an accentuated A_2.

Conversely, A_2 intensity may be diminished in conditions that alter the development of diastolic pressure gradients, such as aortic regurgitation and hypotension. (◆**Sound 9**) A_2 intensity also decreases when ventricular dysfunction is present, such as after an acute myocardial infarction. With this condition, P_2 may become louder if the pulmonary artery pressure rises and systemic pressure falls. A_2 is also softer or absent when aortic valve motion is restricted, as in severe aortic stenosis.

Abnormal S_2 splits

Abnormal splitting is related to valvular dysfunction to alterations in blood flow to or from the ventricles, or to both. These changes may cause the normal S_2 split to be absent during both phases of the respiratory cycle. Thus, only a single S_2 is heard over Erb's point. In another case, the split sounds may persist through inspiration and expiration with little or no respiratory variation. (◆**Sound 10**) The split sounds may also be heard paradoxically on expiration. The A_2-P_2 intervals vary, as does the intensity of A_2 and P_2 during the respiratory cycle. (◆**Sound 11**) Changes in S_2 splits are usually most noticeable at the beginning of inspiration and expiration. (See *PCG and ECG showing abnormal S_2 split with no respiratory variation in a patient with elevated pulmonary artery diastolic pressure and PCG and ECG showing abnormal S_2 split during respiratory cycle,* page 32.)

Absent S_2 split

The P_2 component may not be heard during auscultation over Erb's point in the patient with severe pulmonic stenosis. Consequently, S_2 remains a single sound during both inspiration and expiration. A normal S_2 split may also be absent if the A_2 sound masks the P_2 sound or vice versa—for example, when one sound is significantly louder than the other, making splitting inaudible. This phenomenon occurs in patients with pulmonary hypertension. On the other hand, systemic hypertension causes A_2 to be delayed and to fuse with P_2 during inspiration. In patients with an increased anteroposterior chest dimension, the P_2 intensity may be so diminished that only A_2 is audible.

Persistent S_2 split

A persistent S_2 split occurs when A_2 and P_2 don't fuse into one sound during expiration, even though some respiratory variation in the intensity of A_2 and P_2 is heard. (◆**Sound 12**) This persistent A_2-P_2 splitting during expiration usually results from early aortic valve closure or delayed pulmonic valve closure.

PCG and ECG showing abnormal S₂ split with no respiratory variation in a patient with elevated pulmonary artery diastolic pressure

PCG and ECG showing abnormal S₂ splits during respiratory cycle

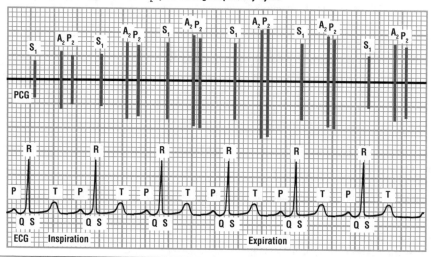

PCG and ECG showing persistent S₂ split

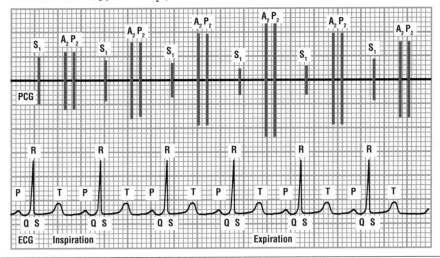

Early aortic valve closure is associated with shortened left ventricular systole, which occurs in patients with mitral regurgitation, ventricular septal defects, or cardiac tamponade. Delayed pulmonic valve closure occurs when right ventricular systole is prolonged in patients with chronic pulmonary hypertension. In these patients, the A_2-P_2 split persists through inspiration and expiration; however, the interval between the A_2 and P_2 components is narrower than it is in a persistent S_2 split (see *PCG and ECG showing narrowed S_2 split in a patient with chronic pulmonary hypertension,* page 34). (◆**Sound 13**)

Delayed electrical activation of the right ventricle
Another cause of persistent A_2-P_2 splitting throughout expiration is the delayed electrical activation of the right ventricle, which will delay P_2. This phenomenon is commonly found in patients with right bundle branch block, left ventricular epicardial pacing, or left ventricular ectopic beats.

PCG and ECG showing narrowed S₂ split in a patient with chronic pulmonary hypertension

PCG and ECG showing wide, fixed S₂ split

Wide, fixed S₂ split

A prolonged right ventricular ejection time produces expiratory A_2-P_2 splits that are widened and that persist even when the patient is seated. (◆Sound 14) This occurs in patients with atrial septal defects, acute pulmonary hypertension secondary to massive pulmonary emboli, or pulmonic stenosis. The P_2 component may not be audible in patients with severe pulmonic stenosis.

A wide, fixed S_2 split is also associated with the pulmonary vascular bed's increased capacitance (ability to receive blood

PCG and ECG showing paradoxical S₂ split during expiration

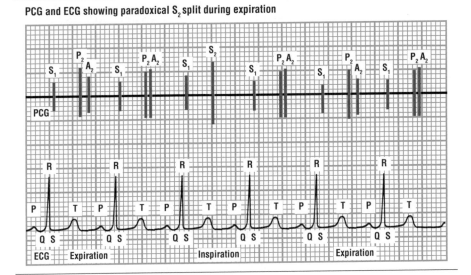

volume and the decreased resistance that accompanies it). (◆**Sound 14**) This phenomenon occurs in patients with idiopathic dilation of the pulmonary artery or with atrial septal defects. This split does not change with respiration.

Paradoxical S₂ split

In a paradoxical, or reversed, S_2 split, P_2 precedes A_2, and the split sounds are heard during expiration instead of inspiration. (◆**Sound 11**) Delayed aortic valve closure almost always causes this phenomenon. If A_2 is delayed during expiration, it may follow P_2, causing an S_2 split; if A_2 is delayed during inspiration, A_2 and P_2 fuse because inspiration normally delays P_2. Therefore, S_2 is heard as a single sound during inspiration instead of a normally split sound. (◆**Sound 15**)

Delayed A_2 is commonly seen in patients with delayed activation of the left ventricle caused by left bundle branch block. It is also associated with right ventricular ectopic beats and with right ventricular endocardial pacing. Prolonged left ventricular systole can also cause a delay in A_2. The same paradoxical P_2-A_2 split may be heard in patients with left-sided heart failure, patent ductus arteriosus, coarctation of the aorta, tricuspid regurgitation, ischemic heart disease, or early right ventricular activation across accessory tracks, as in Wolff–Parkinson–White syndrome.

Left ventricular pressure overload, which occurs in patients with systemic hypertension or hypertrophic cardiomyopathy, may also cause paradoxical S_2 split. Likewise, aortic stenosis may lead to paradoxical splitting of A_2 and P_2; however, if the stenosis is severe, the A_2 component may be inaudible.

With left ventricular volume overload, which is commonly associated with aortic regurgitation or patent ductus arteriosus, A_2 may be delayed, and a paradoxical S_2 split may be heard; however, this is rather uncommon.

◀◀◀POSTTEST

1. What produces S_2?
2. What are the two basic components of S_2?
3. Where is S_2 heard best during auscultation?
4. Describe the characteristics of S_2.
5. How does respiration affect S_2?
6. Describe an abnormal S_2 split.
7. How do severe pulmonic stenosis and pulmonary hypertension affect the S_2 split?
8. Describe a persistent S_2 split.
9. Describe a wide, fixed S_2 split.
10. Describe a paradoxical S_2 split.

CHAPTER 5

The third and fourth heart sounds

PRETEST ▸▸▸

1. Describe a normal S_3.
2. Describe an abnormal S_3 and a right-sided S_3.
3. What is a ventricular gallop, or gallop rhythm?
4. Describe a normal S_4.
5. Describe an abnormal S_4, a summation gallop, and a right-sided S_4.

VENTRICULAR FILLING SOUNDS

The first and second heart sounds, S_1 and S_2, mark the beginning and end, respectively, of ventricular systole. In healthy individuals, these two sounds and their components are relatively easy to hear during auscultation and are best heard with the diaphragm of the stethoscope.

The two left ventricular diastolic filling sounds, S_3 and S_4, are sometimes heard over the mitral area. These sounds differ from S_1 and S_2 in that they're low-frequency sounds produced by ventricular filling, rather than associated with valve closure.

THIRD HEART SOUND

Normal S_3

Occasionally, a physiologic third heart sound, S_3, is heard during auscultation. This heart sound, considered normal in healthy individuals younger than age 20 and in athletic young adults, is caused by vibrations occurring during rapid, passive ventricular filling.

 AGE ISSUE *In patients older than age 40, an S_3 is likely the result of heart failure or ventricular volume overload caused by valvular disease.*

Early in diastole, after isovolumic relaxation, the mitral and tricuspid valves open and the ventricles fill and expand. In children and young adults, the left ventricle is normally compliant, permitting rapid filling. The left ventricle responds to this rapid filling with an abrupt change in wall motion that causes a sudden decrease in blood flow. These events generate vibrations that are responsible for the physiologic S_3. The more vigorously the left ventricle expands, the greater the likelihood that an S_3 will occur.

Area producing S_3

1. Mitral valve
2. Left ventricle
3. Tricuspid valve

PCG and ECG showing physiologic S₃

Auscultatory area for S₃

Mitral area

A physiologic S_3 is also commonly audible in patients with high-output conditions in which rapid ventricular expansion, caused by increased blood volume, is present. Anemia, fever, pregnancy, and thyrotoxicosis are conditions that cause rapid ventricular expansion, resulting in an S_3. An S_3 is also commonly heard in young, slender individuals during periods of excessive catecholamine release.

Auscultatory area and relationship to ECG

S_3 is typically heard best with the bell of the stethoscope over the mitral area, and it can usually be palpated over the same area. It's heard best during expiration when blood flow into the left ventricle is increased. (◆**Sound 16**) S_3 is heard early in diastole and follows S_2 by 0.14 to 0.20 seconds. The relationship of S_3 to the electrocardiogram (ECG) waveform can be seen easily on a phonocardiogram (PCG). In the ECG, S_3 occurs during the T-P interval just after the T wave. Normally, the S_2-S_3 interval is reliably constant.

Sound characteristics

S_3 is usually heard best near the apex of the heart, over the mitral area. In some patients, it's soft and faint in intensity and difficult to hear. In others, it may be loud and easy to hear. S_3 has a short duration, and it may occur only intermittently during every third or fourth heartbeat.

S_3 has a low pitch that's heard best with the bell of the stethoscope. It usually has a dull, thudlike quality. Its timing is closely

PCG and ECG showing abnormal S₃ in a patient older than age 20 with a clinical condition

related to S_2, which is heard just after the T wave. S_3 follows S_2 by less than 0.20 seconds. (◆**Sound 16**)

Enhancing S₃

Because S_3 is associated with blood volume and velocity, it can be intensified by maneuvers that increase stroke volume such as elevating the patient's legs from a recumbent position or having the patient exercise briefly or cough several times. A physiologic S_3 usually disappears with maneuvers that decrease the venous return, such as having the patient sit up or stand.

 AUSCULTATION TIP *To enhance your ability to auscultate and palpate for an S₃, place the patient in a partial left lateral recumbent position.*

Abnormal S₃

The S_1, S_2, S_3 sequence is referred to as a *ventricular gallop* or *gallop rhythm.* (◆**Sound 17**) An abnormal S_3 has the same sound characteristics, is heard over the same location, and has the same timing in relation to S_2 as a physiologic S_3. The differences between the two are related to the patient's age, clinical condition, or both. Also, an S_3 gallop rhythm usually persists despite maneuvers that decrease the venous return. (◆**Sound 17**)

An abnormal S_3 is heard in conditions associated with increased blood volume and increased inflow velocity into the left ventricle. It is heard with or without an increase in ventricular diastolic pressure. Consequently, patients with mitral regurgitation and heart failure have an abnormal S_3. This heart sound can also be heard during increased blood flow through the mitral valve.

Area producing abnormal S₃

1. Mitral valve
2. Thickened left ventricle
3. Tricuspid valve

PCG and ECG showing pericardial knock

Auscultatory area for pericardial knock

1. Third intercostal space
2. Fourth intercostal space
3. Fifth intercostal space

Area producing right-sided S₃

1. Mitral valve
2. Tricuspid valve
3. Right ventricle

This occurs in patients with a ventricular septal defect, patent ductus arteriosus, or severe aortic regurgitation.

AGE ISSUE *The left ventricle becomes less compliant with age. Decreased ventricular compliance leads to pressure changes that cause slowed left ventricular isovolumic relaxation and reduced blood flow velocity into the ventricle. Thus, an audible S_3 in a patient older than age 20 is considered abnormal unless the individual is a highly trained athlete.*

An abnormal S_3 in patients with constrictive pericarditis is called a *pericardial knock*. This type of abnormal S_3 occurs closer to S_2. The interval between S_2 and S_3 is usually less than 0.14 seconds. (**◆Sound 18**) The pericardial knock is easier to hear than a physiologic or abnormal S_3 and is heard best over the third, fourth, and fifth intercostal spaces along the left sternal border using the diaphragm of the stethoscope. (**◆Sound 18**) Inspiration usually intensifies the pericardial knock.

AUSCULTATION TIP *To increase the intensity of an abnormal S_3, have the patient perform maneuvers that increase the venous return to the heart such as raising the legs while in a recumbent position.*

Right-sided S₃
Because the right ventricle is normally much more compliant than the left ventricle, its filling shouldn't cause the vibrations that would create a right-sided S_3. However, in some patients, an S_3 originates in the right ventricle instead of the left. When it does, it is always considered abnormal. (**◆Sound 19**)

PCG and ECG showing right-sided S₃

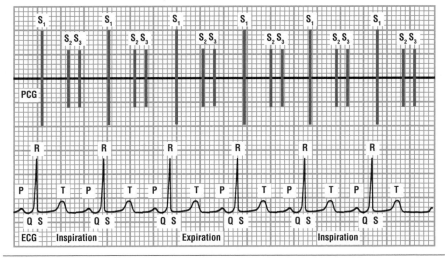

A right-sided S_3 is heard best over the third, fourth, and fifth intercostal spaces along the left sternal border and over the epigastric area. It's more prominent during inspiration because of increased blood flow into the right ventricle. (See *PCG and ECG showing right-sided S_3.*)

Many patients with an enlarged right ventricle have a right-sided S_3. This heart sound is audible in patients with right-sided heart failure, pulmonic regurgitation, or severe tricuspid insufficiency. (◆**Sound 19**)

FOURTH HEART SOUND

Normal S_4

By the end of diastole, the ventricles are nearly full; atrial contraction further stretches and fills the ventricles. The vibrations caused by this filling and stretching in late diastole generate an additional fourth heart sound, S_4, sometimes called an *atrial diastolic gallop*. (◆**Sound 20**) An S_4 is usually abnormal except in highly trained young athletes with physiologic left ventricular hypertrophy.

Because S_4 is associated with atrial contraction, it isn't produced in conditions in which atrial systole doesn't occur, such as atrial fibrillation.

Auscultatory area and relationship to ECG

S_4 is usually heard best with the bell of the stethoscope during expiration near the heart's apex over the mitral area. It may also be palpable in this area. The relationship of S_4 to S_1 can be seen

Auscultatory area for right-sided S₃

1. Third intercostal space
2. Fourth intercostal space
3. Fifth intercostal space
4. Epigastric area

PCG and ECG showing S₄

Area producing S₄

1. Mitral valve
2. Left ventricle

Auscultatory area for S₄

Mitral area

easily on the ECG waveform: S_4 occurs during the P-R interval and precedes S_1.

Sound characteristics

S_4 is usually located near the heart's apex over the mitral area. Occasionally, it is also palpable over this area. In some patients, it is faint in intensity and difficult to hear. In others, it is loud and easy to hear. S_4 is relatively short in duration and may occur only intermittently during every third or fourth heartbeat. It has a low pitch and a thudlike quality that is heard best with the bell of the stethoscope. The timing is presystolic: S_4 precedes S_1 and occurs during the P-R interval. (◆**Sound 20**)

 AUSCULTATION TIP *To enhance S_4, place the patient in the partial left lateral recumbent position, which brings the heart closer to the chest wall.*

Abnormal S₄

An abnormal S_4 is usually associated with increased mean left atrial pressure caused by a noncompliant left ventricle. This auscultatory finding is heard in patients with hypertension (the most common cause), hypertrophic cardiomyopathy, or ischemic heart disease; during an episode of angina; and during or after an acute myocardial infarction. When an S_4 is heard in a patient with hypertension, the systolic blood pressure usually exceeds 160 mm Hg or the diastolic pressure exceeds 100 mm Hg.

An abnormal S_4 can also accompany certain volume overload conditions, such as hyperthyroidism, certain anemias, and sudden severe mitral regurgitation.

 AGE ISSUE *In children, an S_4 may accompany congenital abnormalities associated with heart failure, such as a large ventricular septal defect and patent ductus arteriosus. It may also result from sickle cell anemia.*

Summation gallop

Normally, S_4 precedes S_1 by an appreciable interval that correlates with the P-R interval on the ECG. However, in patients with first-degree atrioventricular block, the P wave occurs early in diastole, and S_4 may occur during the early rapid diastolic filling period. Likewise, with tachycardia, S_4 may be superimposed on S_3 during early rapid filling. If either condition exists, the S_4 fuses with S_3 to become a single diastolic filling sound called a *summation gallop*, which may be louder than S_4, S_3, or S_1. (**◆Sound 21**)

Right-sided S_4

An S_4 generated in the right ventricle is called a *right-sided S4*. (**◆Sound 22**) It's commonly heard in patients with conditions that increase pressure in the right ventricle by more than 100 mm Hg, such as pulmonic stenosis or pulmonary hypertension. This heart sound is heard best over the third, fourth, and fifth intercostal spaces along the left sternal border and over the epigastric area, with the patient in a supine position. It is more audible during inspiration.

Differentiating S_4 from an S_1 split

Distinguishing an S_1 split (M_1-T_1) from an S_4-S_1 sequence is sometimes difficult. There are, however, some ways to help you do so. Here are some tips. First, an S_1 split is heard best between the mitral and tricuspid areas with the diaphragm of the stethoscope in comparison to an S_4 that is heard best over the mitral area with the bell of the stethoscope. An S_4 may also be palpable.

 AUSCULTATION TIP *To increase the intensity of S_4, have the patient perform maneuvers that increase left atrial pressure, such as the handgrip exercise.*

S_3 AND S_4: SIMILARITIES AND DIFFERENCES

S_3, like S_4, is low-pitched and may be faint or loud and heard only intermittently. Both sounds are heard best over the mitral area using the bell of the stethoscope, with the patient in a partial left lateral recumbent position. Both sounds are intensified by expiration and can be enhanced by maneuvers that increase stroke volume, such as elevating the legs while in a recumbent position or performing handgrip exercises.

Area producing right-sided S_4

1. Mitral valve
2. Tricuspid valve
3. Right ventricle

Auscultatory area for right-sided S_4

1. Third intercostal space
2. Fourth intercostal space
3. Fifth intercostal space
4. Epigastric area

PCG and ECG showing summation gallop

PCG and ECG showing right-sided S₄

◀◀◀ POSTTEST

1. How is an S_3 produced?
2. Where and when is S_3 heard best?
3. Describe the characteristics of S_3.
4. Which maneuvers can be used to enhance S_3?
5. Describe the characteristics of a right-sided S_3.
6. How is an S_4 produced?
7. Describe the characteristics of S_4.
8. How can an S_4 be enhanced?
9. In which conditions is an abnormal S_4 heard?
10. Describe a summation gallop.

3

Abnormal heart sounds

CHAPTER 6

Other diastolic and systolic sounds

PRETEST ▶▶▶

1. What causes an opening snap?
2. How can you differentiate an opening snap from a second or a third heart sound (S_2 or S_3)?
3. What is the difference between a pulmonic ejection sound and an aortic ejection sound?
4. What is a midsystolic click (MSC)?
5. How can you differentiate an MSC from other heart sounds?

Area producing opening snap

Narrowed
mitral valve

OPENING SNAPS

At the end of ventricular systole, the aortic and pulmonic valves close, generating the second heart sound, S_2. S_2 is followed by a brief period of isovolumic relaxation; during this time, ventricular pressures fall. When ventricular pressures are less than atrial pressures, the mitral and tricuspid valves open. Normally, the opening of these heart valves is inaudible. However, if the mitral valve leaflets become stenotic or abnormally narrowed while remaining somewhat mobile, they create an *opening snap* (OS). (◆**Sound 23**) The OS sound is generated by the maximum, but limited, opening of the stenotic leaflets and usually indicates the beginning of the diastolic murmur associated with mitral stenosis. If the mitral valve becomes severely calcified and inflexible, the OS disappears. If the tricuspid valve leaflets become stenotic or abnormally narrowed, an OS can be produced.

Auscultatory area and relationship to ECG

An OS is heard best with the diaphragm of the stethoscope near the heart's apex over the mitral area or just medial to it, with the patient in the left lateral decubitus position. It's transmitted widely across the precordium and can typically be heard over the aortic, pulmonic, and tricuspid areas as well. An OS is higher in pitch than S_2; it may be as loud as or louder than S_2.

An OS occurs early in ventricular diastole; thus, it's heard just after the T wave in the electrocardiogram (ECG) waveform.

PCG and ECG showing opening snap

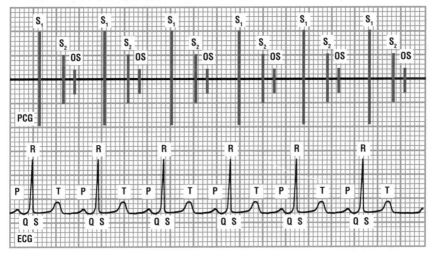

Sound characteristics

The intensity of an OS varies among patients, and it's usually easy to hear during auscultation. An OS has a short duration. It has a high pitch that's heard best with the diaphragm of the stethoscope, and a sharp, snaplike quality. Its timing is closely related to S_2; an OS occurs early in ventricular diastole, just after the stenotic mitral valve opens. (**♦Sound 23**)

Differentiating an OS from S_2

An OS occurs early in diastole and consequently may be confused with P_2 or S_3. One characteristic of an OS that helps distinguish it from P_2 is its timing: the A_2-P_2 interval is normally shorter than the A_2-OS interval. Also, when the patient stands, the A_2-P_2 interval narrows, whereas the A_2-OS interval widens.

Another characteristic is that the A_2-OS interval remains constant throughout respiration, whereas the A_2-P_2 interval normally widens during inspiration and narrows during expiration. During inspiration, three distinct sounds can usually be heard over the pulmonic area; therefore, the sequence must be A_2, P_2, OS. In contrast, during expiration, the A_2-P_2 interval narrows or fuses, forming one sound. This creates an S_2-OS interval.

Finally, P_2 isn't usually heard over the mitral area. Therefore, if you hear a split S_2 over this area, it may be an S_2 and an OS.

Auscultatory area for opening snap

Mitral area

Differentiating an OS from S₃

Distinguishing an OS from an S_3 is difficult in some patients, especially in those with mild mitral stenosis when the A_2-OS interval is wider than usual and the OS is somewhat softer. One characteristic of an OS that helps distinguish it from an S_3 is its timing: the A_2-S_3 interval is usually longer than the A_2-OS interval. Also, S_3 is a low-frequency sound that's heard best over the mitral area using the bell of the stethoscope. In contrast, an OS produces a high-frequency sound that's more widely transmitted across the precordium and heard best using the diaphragm of the stethoscope.

Another characteristic of an OS is that its intensity usually isn't affected by having the patient stand, whereas S_2 intensity can be decreased by standing. If the OS is affected, it's intensified. Finally, if the murmur typically heard in patients with mitral stenosis is present, you can confirm that the sound is an OS.

 AUSCULTATION TIP *S_3 is usually louder during expiration than during inspiration and is typically palpable; an OS doesn't vary in intensity with respiration.*

SYSTOLIC EJECTION SOUNDS

Just as an OS is caused by stenotic mitral valve leaflets, a systolic ejection sound (ES) is caused by the opening of a stenotic aortic or pulmonic valve.

A systolic ES usually occurs early in systole after S_1 and isovolumic contraction. It's commonly associated with ventricular ejection and the maximum opening of a stenotic, yet mobile, aortic or pulmonic valve. If the valve is severely stenotic because of calcification, a systolic ES—like an OS—won't be produced.

A systolic ES is considered an abnormal condition, regardless of whether it originates on the heart's right or left side. It may also be caused by the sudden distention of an already dilated aorta or pulmonary artery and by forceful ventricular ejection from pulmonary or systemic hypertension.

Auscultatory area and relationship to ECG

A systolic ES is usually a brief, high-frequency sound that's heard best using the diaphragm of the stethoscope. It may be heard near the heart's base over the aortic or pulmonic area, over Erb's point, or near the apex over the mitral area. A systolic ES occurs just after the QRS complex on the ECG waveform.

Area producing ejection sound

Stenotic aortic or pulmonic valve

Pulmonic ejection sounds

A pulmonic ejection sound (PES), heard best over the pulmonic area, is the only right-sided heart sound that increases in intensity during expiration and diminishes or disappears during inspiration. (◆**Sound 24**) In a normal heart, inspiration increases the right ventricular volume, causing the pulmonic valve to dome toward the pulmonary artery, which decreases the sound's intensity. During expiration, the right ventricular volume is decreased, the valve is less domed, and its opening produces a louder snap. In a patient with pulmonary artery dilation or pulmonary hypertension, a PES may not vary in intensity during respiration.

Auscultatory area for pulmonic ejection sound

Pulmonic area

Sound characteristics

A PES is usually heard best near the base of the heart over the pulmonic area. Its intensity is soft but may be equal to or greater than that of S_1; it has a short duration. It has a high pitch that is heard best with the diaphragm of the stethoscope and a sharp, or clicklike, quality. Its timing is closely related to S_1. A PES occurs early in ventricular systole, just after the opening of a stenotic pulmonic valve (◆**Sound 24**), and is heard just after the QRS complex. (See *PCG and ECG showing pulmonic ejection sound*, page 52.)

AUSCULTATION TIP *To differentiate between a PES and an S_1, remember that a PES is heard in the pulmonic area and varies with respiration, whereas a split S_1 is heard in the tricuspid area and does not vary with respiration.*

PCG and ECG showing pulmonic ejection sound

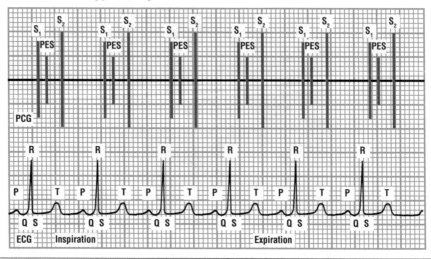

Auscultatory area for aortic ejection sound

1. Aortic area
2. Erb's point
3. Mitral area

Using a PES to differentiate clinical conditions

Because a PES may occur in idiopathic dilation of the pulmonary artery, but usually isn't present in supravalvular or muscular subvalvular obstructions, its presence can be used to differentiate between these conditions. Occasionally, a PES may also be heard with atrial and ventricular septal defects.

Aortic ejection sounds

An aortic ejection sound (AES) is heard best near the heart's apex over the mitral area, near the heart's base over the aortic area, or over Erb's point. An AES may be heard in patients with aortic stenosis or aortic insufficiency, but the sound is less clicklike when associated with aortic insufficiency. (◆**Sound 25**)

Unlike a PES, caused by pulmonic valve stenosis, an AES, caused by aortic valve stenosis, doesn't vary in intensity with respiration. An AES may occur in patients with aortic root dilation, which is commonly associated with such conditions as systemic hypertension, an ascending aortic aneurysm, or coarctation of the aorta.

Sound characteristics

An AES is heard best near the heart's apex over the mitral area, near the heart's base over the aortic area, or over Erb's point. Having the patient sit up and lean forward facilitates auscultation. Its intensity is soft but may be equal to or greater than that of S_1 (to distinguish it from a split S_2, ask the patient to take a deep breath and hold it). An AES has a short duration. It has a high pitch that's heard best using the diaphragm of the stethoscope and a sharp, or clicklike, quality. Its timing is closely related to S_1.

PCG and ECG showing aortic ejection sound

(◆**Sound 25**) An AES occurs early in ventricular systole, just after the opening of a stenotic aortic valve, and is heard just after the QRS complex in the ECG waveform.

Differentiating an AES from other heart sounds

Certain characteristics help to distinguish an AES from other heart sounds. One characteristic is that an AES radiates more than a PES. Another characteristic is that a split S_1 heard over the mitral area is likely to be an M_1 and an AES.

You can differentiate an AES from an S_4 by remembering that S_4 is heard best over the mitral area using the bell of the stethoscope and is commonly accompanied by a palpable, presystolic apical bulge. Also, an S_4 is intensified by maneuvers that increase left atrial pressure, such as brief exercise, squatting, or coughing. An AES is unaffected by these maneuvers.

Clicks

A midsystolic click (MSC) occurs when the prolapsed mitral valve's leaflets and chordae tendineae tense. The anterior leaflet, the posterior leaflet, or both can prolapse, causing a balloon backup into the left atrium. Occasionally, multiple clicks occur that are heard in midsystole to late systole; they're heard best over the tricuspid area and toward the mitral area. Like ESs, these midsystolic to late systolic clicks are crisp, high-frequency sounds. (◆**Sound 26**)

Area producing midsystolic click

1. Enlarged leaflets
2. Normal mitral valve position

PCG and ECG showing midsystolic click

Auscultatory area for midsystolic click

1. Tricuspid area
2. Mitral area

Sound characteristics

An MSC is usually heard best over the tricuspid area and near the heart's apex over the mitral area. Its intensity is equal to or greater than that of S_1. An MSC has a short duration. It has a high pitch that's heard best using the diaphragm of the stethoscope, and its quality is clicklike. The click's timing varies; it can occur in early systole, midsystole, or late systole. An MSC can be heard during the Q-T interval in the ECG waveform. (◆Sound 26)

Differentiating an MSC from other heart sounds

The timing of an MSC is affected by various maneuvers, such as having the patient stand or perform the Valsalva's maneuver. Such maneuvers result in reduced left ventricular filling and cause the MSC to be heard closer to S_1. The MSC may even merge with S_1 and disappear completely. Increasing the left ventricular volume by raising the legs from a recumbent position or squatting delays the click. This maneuver may also cause the prolapse not to occur and the MSC to be diminished or inaudible.

Sometimes an MSC is accompanied by a late systolic crescendo murmur, as in mitral valve prolapse, or the characteristic holosystolic murmur, as in mitral regurgitation. An MSC may also be caused by some extracardiac conditions, such as pleuropericardial adhesions, atrial septal aneurysms, and cardiac tumors.

◀◀◀POSTTEST

1. Describe the characteristics of an OS.
2. How can you tell the difference between an OS and S_2?
3. How can you tell the difference between an OS and S_3?
4. What is a systolic ejection sound?
5. Describe the characteristics of a PES.
6. Describe the characteristics of an AES.
7. How can you tell the difference between an AES and other heart sounds?
8. What causes an MSC?
9. Describe the characteristics of an MSC.
10. How can you tell the difference between an MSC and other heart sounds?

Murmur fundamentals

PRETEST ◆◆◆

1. How does turbulent blood flow produce murmurs?
2. What are the seven characteristics used to describe murmurs?
3. What is the six-point graded scale?
4. What is a murmur's configuration?

TURBULENT BLOOD FLOW

Whereas heart sounds are produced by brief vibrations that correspond to the beginning and end of systole, murmurs are produced by a prolonged series of vibrations that occurs during systole, diastole, or both. These vibrations result from turbulent blood flow.

Several clinically significant conditions—such as blood flowing at a high velocity through a partially obstructed opening, blood flowing from a higher-pressure chamber to a lower-pressure one, or any combination of these—can cause turbulent blood flow.

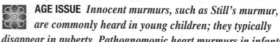 **AGE ISSUE** *Innocent murmurs, such as Still's murmur, are commonly heard in young children; they typically disappear in puberty. Pathognomonic heart murmurs in infants and young children usually result from congenital heart disease, such as atrial and ventricular septal defects. Other murmurs heard in pediatric patients can be acquired, such as with rheumatic heart disease.*

CHARACTERISTICS

Murmurs, like other heart sounds, are described by their audible characteristics identified during auscultation. The terms used to describe a specific characteristic are determined primarily by the volume and speed of the jet of blood as it moves through the heart.

The seven characteristics used to describe murmurs are location, intensity, duration, pitch, quality, timing, and configuration.

AUSCULTATION TIP *Initially, learn to identify the location and timing of murmurs. As your auscultation techniques improve, try to identify the intensity, duration, pitch, quality, and configuration.*

AGE ISSUE *When listening to heart sounds in the pediatric patient, take into account that exercise, crying, fever, and position changes can accentuate murmurs.*

Location

A murmur's location is the anatomic area on the chest wall where the murmur is heard best and is usually also the murmur's point of maximum intensity. This area usually correlates with the underlying location of the valve that's responsible for producing the murmur. For example, an aortic stenosis murmur is usually heard best near the heart's base over the aortic area, whereas a mitral regurgitation murmur is usually heard best near the heart's apex over the mitral area.

The murmur's sounds may also be transmitted to the chamber or vessel where the turbulent blood flow occurs. This phenomenon, known as *radiation*, occurs because the direction of blood flow determines sound transmission. Murmurs radiate in either a forward or a backward direction.

Intensity

Intensity refers to a murmur's loudness. It's influenced by many factors, including body weight. For example, because the transmission of heart sounds to the chest wall is affected by chest wall thickness and by certain diseases, heart sounds and murmurs are usually louder in thin individuals and fainter in obese individuals. They're also fainter in patients with emphysema.

Hyperdynamic states, decreased blood viscosity, increased pressure gradients across valves, larger jets of blood, and faster heart rates may also increase a murmur's intensity. Murmurs are less intense in hypodynamic states and in patients with an elevated hematocrit.

Documenting intensity

Document a murmur's intensity using a uniform method. Most health care professionals use a six-point graded scale, with 1 being the faintest intensity and 6 being the loudest. A grade 1 murmur is faint, may be heard intermittently, and is barely heard through the stethoscope. A grade 2 murmur is also faint but is usually heard as soon as the stethoscope is placed on the chest wall. A grade 3 murmur is easily heard and is described as moderately loud. A grade 4 murmur is loud and is usually associated with a palpable vibration known as a *thrill*. It may also radiate in the direction of blood flow. A grade 5 murmur is loud enough to be heard with only an edge of the stethoscope touching the chest wall; it's almost always accompanied by a thrill and radiation. A grade 6 murmur is so loud that it can be heard with the stethoscope close to, but not touching, the chest wall; it's always accompanied by a thrill, and it radiates to distant structures. Both grade 5 and 6 may even be heard without the aid of a stethoscope.

When you document a murmur's grade, write it as a fraction—for example, 3/6. This means you consider it to be a grade 3 and have used the six-point scale for assessment. That way, all health care professionals will understand which scale was used, even if they don't use the same one.

Duration

A murmur's duration is the length of time the murmur is heard during systole or diastole. It is described as long or short.

Pitch

A murmur's pitch, or frequency, varies from high-pitched to low-pitched. It's usually higher in conditions accompanied by increased blood flow velocity or increased pressure gradients and lower in conditions associated with lower blood flow velocity. High-pitched sounds are best heard with the diaphragm of the stethoscope and low-pitched sounds are best heard with the bell of the stethoscope.

Quality

A murmur's quality is determined by the combination of frequencies that produces the sound. It's typically described as harsh, rough, musical, scratchy, squeaky, rumbling, or blowing.

Timing

A murmur's timing refers to when the murmur occurs in the cardiac cycle. This means that the onset, duration, and end of the murmur are described in relation to systole and diastole. The beginning of systole, or the first heart sound (S_1), can be identified easily by palpating the carotid pulse or by looking for the QRS complex on the electrocardiogram (ECG) monitor's oscilloscope.

All systolic murmurs occur between S_1 and the second heart sound (S_2) during ventricular systole; this interval is between the QRS complex and the T wave in the ECG waveform. All diastolic murmurs occur between S_2 and S_1 during ventricular diastole; this interval is between the T wave and the QRS complex in the ECG waveform.

Murmurs are further classified according to their timing within the phases of the cardiac cycle. For example, a murmur can be described as holosystolic, meaning it's present throughout systole; early systolic, midsystolic, or late systolic; or early diastolic, mid-diastolic, or late diastolic.

Configuration

A murmur's configuration refers to the shape of a murmur's sound as recorded on a phonocardiogram. The configuration is usually defined by changes in the murmur's intensity during systole or diastole and is determined by blood flow pressure gradients. For example, a *crescendo murmur* is one that gradually increases in intensity as the pressure gradient increases. A *decrescendo murmur* is one that gradually decreases in intensity as the pressure gradient decreases. A *crescendo–decrescendo murmur* first increases in intensity as the pressure gradient increases, then decreases in intensity as the pressure gradient decreases; it's also

Murmur's configuration

Crescendo murmur

Decrescendo murmur

Crescendo–decrescendo murmur

Plateau-shaped murmur

known as a *diamond-shaped murmur*. Finally, a *plateau-shaped murmur* is one that's equal in intensity throughout the murmur.

Putting them all together

Murmurs must be described carefully and accurately using these seven characteristics. Making such information immediately available to all who care for a specific patient allows any changes in a murmur's characteristics to be recognized easily. In that way, the possible source of those changes can be assessed more easily.

◀◀◀ POSTTEST

1. What determines a murmur's sound characteristics?
2. What is a murmur's location?
3. What does the term *radiation* mean?
4. What is a murmur's intensity?
5. Describe the six-point graded scale.
6. What is a murmur's duration?
7. What is a murmur's pitch?
8. What is a murmur's quality?
9. What is a murmur's timing?
10. What is a murmur's configuration?

Systolic murmurs

CHAPTER 8

PRETEST ◆◆◆

1. How is the sound of a systolic murmur produced?
2. List the murmurs associated with right ventricular outflow obstruction.
3. List the murmurs associated with left ventricular outflow obstruction.
4. How is the sound of a systolic regurgitation murmur produced?
5. List the systolic regurgitation murmurs.

ANATOMY AND PHYSIOLOGY

Normally, as ventricular pressures rise at the beginning of systole, the mitral and tricuspid valves close. For a brief time, while the aortic and pulmonic valves are still closed during isovolumic contraction, ventricular pressures rise sharply. When the pressure in both ventricles is high enough, the aortic and pulmonic valves open, and blood is ejected from the ventricles into the aorta and the pulmonary artery. Normally functioning valves facilitate this unidirectional blood flow.

However, aortic or pulmonic outlet abnormalities may generate forward systolic ejection murmurs. When the mitral or tricuspid valve is involved, backward, or *regurgitant*, murmurs may be heard during systole. All systolic murmurs occur during ventricular systole between the first and second heart sounds (S_1 and S_2).

AGE ISSUE *Between ages 30 and 80, the left ventricular wall grows 25% thicker from its increased efforts to pump blood. Heart valves also become thicker from fibrotic and sclerotic changes. This thickening can prevent the valves from closing completely, causing systolic murmurs.*

SYSTOLIC EJECTION MURMURS

During ventricular systole, the rapid ejection of blood from the ventricles causes turbulent blood flow, which produces an innocent systolic ejection murmur (SEM). (◆**Sound 27**) This murmur, which is considered to be normal, is usually inaudible. However, in thin-chested individuals, children, and patients with hyperdynamic states, such as anemia, thyrotoxicosis, fever, pregnancy, or arteriovenous shunts, an SEM can usually be auscultated.

Area producing systolic ejection murmur

1. Aortic valve
2. Pulmonic valve
3. Left ventricle
4. Right ventricle

Auscultatory area for systolic ejection murmur

Aortic area

Left sternal border

Mitral area

An SEM, classified as benign or functional, is called an *innocent* or *flow murmur* because there's no associated physiologic or structural abnormality. However, unusual turbulence related to dilation of the aorta or pulmonary artery may also produce an innocent SEM. Researchers believe SEMs can be caused by sclerotic changes in the aortic valve cusps.

 AGE ISSUE *About 50% of all persons older than age 50 have this type of murmur, which is heard more commonly in women and in patients with hypertension.*

Sound characteristics

An SEM is usually heard best along the left sternal border and sometimes over the aortic and mitral areas. Its intensity is usually soft (less than a grade 3/6), and the duration of the murmur is short.

 AUSCULTATION TIP *To determine if a murmur intensifies, listen at the murmur's border.*

An SEM has a medium pitch that's heard best using the diaphragm of the stethoscope. The quality of an SEM varies. Its timing is early systolic; it ends well before a normal S$_2$ split. It's heard after the QRS complex on the electrocardiogram (ECG) waveform. An SEM has a crescendo–decrescendo configuration. (◆Sound 27)

Enhancement techniques

An SEM's intensity can be increased by maneuvers that increase blood volume or ejection velocity, such as having the patient raise his legs from a recumbent position, exercise briefly, or cough a few times.

PCG and ECG showing systolic ejection murmur

VENTRICULAR OUTFLOW OBSTRUCTION MURMURS

Right or left ventricular outflow obstructions may be supravalvular, valvular, or subvalvular. Regardless of location, the outflow obstruction causes turbulent blood flow, which produces a midsystolic ejection murmur. The murmur begins early in systole—after S_1 and the opening of the diseased pulmonic or aortic valve. It ends before the S_2 closure component of the diseased pulmonic or aortic valve. This murmur typically has a crescendo–decrescendo configuration that peaks in intensity in early systole, midsystole, or late systole, depending on the severity of the obstruction.

Right ventricular outflow obstruction murmurs

Supravalvular pulmonic stenosis murmurs

Supravalvular pulmonic stenosis, or *pulmonary artery branch stenosis*, is a type of right ventricular outflow obstruction that occurs above the pulmonic valve. This obstruction produces a murmur with a crescendo–decrescendo configuration that's occasionally continuous. (◆**Sound 28)** The murmur is rarely accompanied by a pulmonic ejection sound (PES) and is associated with a P_2 of normal intensity.

Area producing supravalvular pulmonic stenosis murmur

Supravalvular pulmonic area

PCG and ECG showing supravalvular pulmonic stenosis murmur

PCG and ECG showing supravalvular pulmonic stenosis murmur

Auscultatory area for supravalvular pulmonic stenosis murmur

Area producing pulmonic valvular stenosis murmur

Pulmonic valvular area

Sound characteristics

A supravalvular pulmonic stenosis murmur is usually heard over much of the thorax. Its intensity and duration vary. It has a medium pitch that's heard best using the diaphragm of the stethoscope, and it has a harsh quality. Its timing is systolic: it begins after S_1 and ends before a normal S_2 split. On the ECG waveform, the murmur begins just after the QRS complex begins and ends just before the T wave ends. It has a crescendo–decrescendo configuration that's occasionally continuous.
(◆Sound 28)

Pulmonic valvular stenosis murmurs

A pulmonic valvular stenosis murmur results from congenital pulmonic valvular stenosis and is commonly associated with other congenital defects. In mild pulmonic valvular stenosis, S_1 is normal. The murmur begins after S_1 with a right-sided PES as the pulmonic valve abruptly stops opening. Remember, the PES is the only right-sided heart sound that increases in intensity during expiration and becomes less audible during inspiration. The murmur intensifies after the PES and peaks in midsystole; then it begins to fade. It ends before S_2. The intensity of P_2 is normal.
(◆Sound 29)

With severe pulmonic valvular stenosis, the pressure gradient across the pulmonic valve increases. An increased pressure gradient causes the PES to be heard earlier; it may even fuse with S_1.

PCG and ECG showing pulmonic valvular stenosis murmur

The right ventricular ejection time is also prolonged. Consequently, the murmur has a longer crescendo and the intensity peaks later in systole. It continues throughout A_2 but ends before P_2. Prolonged right ventricular ejection time also causes a delayed P_2, creating a wide S_2 split.

Usually, as the stenosis becomes more severe, the murmur's duration lengthens and its configuration becomes more asymmetrical. Consequently, P_2 is delayed even more and its intensity is decreased.

Sound characteristics

A pulmonic valvular stenosis murmur is heard best near the heart's base over the pulmonic area. It commonly radiates toward the left side of the neck or the left shoulder. The murmur's intensity is usually soft, but it will become louder with a palpable thrill toward the left side of the neck and the left shoulder as the stenosis becomes more severe. Its duration is short, but this too will increase as the stenosis worsens. It has a medium pitch that's heard best using the diaphragm of the stethoscope and a harsh quality. Its timing is midsystolic: it ends before a normal S_2 split. It's accompanied by a PES that diminishes or disappears with inspiration. On the ECG waveform, it begins after the QRS complex and ends before the T wave ends. The murmur has a crescendo–decrescendo configuration. A mild pulmonic valvular stenosis murmur is shaped like a diamond; a severe pulmonic valvular stenosis murmur, like a kite. (◆**Sound 29**)

Auscultatory area for pulmonic valvular stenosis murmur

Pulmonic area

PCG and ECG showing subvalvular pulmonic stenosis murmur

Area producing subvalvular pulmonic stenosis murmur

Subvalvular pulmonic area

Auscultatory area for subvalvular pulmonic stenosis murmur

1. Pulmonic area
2. Erb's point

Subvalvular pulmonic stenosis murmurs

When a right ventricular outflow obstruction is beneath the pulmonic valve, or subvalvular, the midsystolic ejection murmur sounds the same as a pulmonic valvular stenosis murmur. However, it isn't initiated by a PES. (◆**Sound 30**) If the subvalvular obstruction is associated with a ventricular septal defect, the murmur will be more complex in character.

Sound characteristics

A subvalvular pulmonic stenosis murmur is usually heard best over the pulmonic area and over Erb's point; it commonly radiates toward the left side of the neck, the left shoulder, or both. Its intensity is usually soft but becomes louder as the stenosis worsens. The duration, which is short, also increases as the stenosis worsens. The murmur has a medium pitch that's heard best using the diaphragm of the stethoscope; its quality is harsh. Its timing is midsystolic: it starts after S_1 and ends before a normal S_2 split. On an ECG, the murmur begins after the QRS complex and ends before the T wave ends. (◆**Sound 30**) This murmur isn't initiated by a PES. It has a crescendo–decrescendo configuration.

Left ventricular outflow obstruction murmurs
Supravalvular aortic stenosis murmurs

When a left ventricular outflow obstruction is above the aortic valve, or supravalvular, it produces a murmur with

PCG and ECG showing supravalvular aortic stenosis murmur

a crescendo–decrescendo configuration. Supravalvular aortic stenosis is usually congenital. Its characteristics are similar to those of aortic valvular stenosis, except that it has no aortic ejection sound (AES), is louder, and is heard best over the suprasternal area, aortic area, or right first intercostal space. (◆**Sound 31**)

Sound characteristics

A supravalvular aortic stenosis murmur is usually heard best near the heart's base over the right first intercostal space, over the aortic area, and over the suprasternal notch. It may radiate toward the right side of the neck, the right shoulder, or both. Its intensity, typically a grade $3/6$ to $4/6$, decreases in patients with left-sided heart failure. Its duration increases as the stenosis worsens. It has a medium pitch that can be heard equally well with the diaphragm or bell of the stethoscope. The murmur has a rough quality. Its timing is midsystolic: it ends before a normal S_2 split. It isn't associated with an AES. On the ECG waveform, it begins after the QRS complex and ends before the T wave ends. The murmur has a crescendo–decrescendo configuration. (◆**Sound 31**)

Area producing supravalvular aortic stenosis murmur

Supravalvular aortic area

Auscultatory area for supravalvular aortic stenosis murmur

1. Suprasternal notch
2. First intercostal space
3. Aortic area

Area producing aortic valvular stenosis murmur

Aortic valvular area

Auscultatory area for aortic valvular pulmonic stenosis murmur

1. Suprasternal notch
2. Aortic area
3. Erb's point
4. Mitral area

Aortic valvular stenosis murmurs

Aortic valvular stenosis may be congenital or may be acquired from degenerative or rheumatic heart disease. If it's acquired from rheumatic heart disease, the mitral valve is commonly affected as well. Aortic stenosis produces an SEM that begins after S_1 and ends before S_2. (◆**Sound 32**) After S_1, the left ventricular pressure rises. The stenotic aortic valve halts its opening motion and produces a loud AES that's heard best near the heart's apex over the mitral area. The AES is followed by the murmur, which gradually intensifies until midsystole to late systole and then fades, ending before a faint A_2.

AGE ISSUE *As a person ages, such changes as the development of fibrous tissues, which thicken the bases of the aortic leaflets, and calcification can lead to an aortic systolic murmur. Aortic stenosis develops if the valve leaflets become increasingly stiff and stationary. This is a gradual process that occurs across the life span.*

When an aortic valvular stenosis murmur is discovered late in adulthood, it can be heard best over the mitral area. As the valve becomes more calcified with age—and consequently less mobile—both the AES and A_2 become soft or even inaudible. The murmur can vary in intensity from a soft grade $2/6$ to a rough grade $4/6$ sound, but most aortic valvular stenosis murmurs are a grade $3/6$ to $4/6$.

Sound characteristics

An aortic valvular stenosis murmur is usually heard best near the heart's base over the aortic area, over Erb's point, near the heart's apex over the mitral area, or over the suprasternal notch. The murmur may radiate toward the right side of the neck, the right shoulder, or both. A thrill may be palpable over the aortic area and neck. The murmur's intensity, typically a grade $3/6$ to $4/6$, decreases in patients with left-sided heart failure. Its duration increases as stenosis worsens.

An aortic valvular stenosis murmur has a medium pitch that's heard equally well using the diaphragm or the bell of the stethoscope. The murmur's quality is rough and may become harsher and louder as stenosis worsens. Its timing is midsystolic. An AES, when present, is heard shortly after S_1; the AES is followed by the murmur, which ends before a normal S_2 split. If an S_4 is heard before age 40, stenosis is usually severe. On the ECG waveform, the murmur begins after the QRS complex and ends before the T wave ends. It has a crescendo–decrescendo configuration. (◆**Sound 32**) As the stenosis worsens, valve

PCG and ECG showing aortic valvular stenosis murmur

motion is reduced and the aortic component of the second heart sound disappears.

Variations

Certain characteristics of an aortic valvular stenosis murmur vary according to the degree of stenosis. For example, as stenosis worsens, the left ventricular ejection time is prolonged, and the murmur peaks later in systole. A delayed A_2 and a shortened A_2-P_2 interval are also heard.

Also, the more severe the stenosis, the closer A_2 moves to P_2. With extremely severe stenosis, A_2 becomes soft and actually follows P_2, producing a paradoxical S_2 split.

Subvalvular aortic stenosis murmurs

When a left ventricular outflow obstruction is below the aortic valve, or subvalvular, it produces a murmur with a crescendo–decrescendo configuration. (**◆Sound 33**) A subvalvular aortic outflow obstruction may be caused by a congenital fibrous ring, or it may be acquired from hypertrophic obstructive cardiomyopathy (formerly known as *idiopathic hypertrophic subaortic stenosis*). This is a dynamic obstruction produced by asymmetrical hypertrophy of the septum and an abnormal anterior motion of the mitral valve leaflets during systole.

Area producing subvalvular aortic stenosis murmur

Subvalvular aortic stenosis area

PCG and ECG showing subvalvular aortic stenosis murmur

Sound characteristics

A subvalvular aortic stenosis murmur is usually heard best near the heart's apex over the mitral and tricuspid areas. It doesn't usually radiate toward the base, right side of the neck, or right shoulder. Its intensity, typically a grade 3/6 to 4/6, increases as stenosis worsens; its duration varies. The murmur has a medium pitch that's heard equally well using the bell or the diaphragm of the stethoscope. Its quality can be harsh or rough. This murmur's timing is midsystolic: it peaks in midsystole and ends before a normal S_2 split, a delayed A_2, or a paradoxical S_2 split. On the ECG waveform, it begins after the QRS complex and ends before the T wave ends. The murmur has a crescendo–decrescendo configuration. (◆**Sound 33**)

Differentiating subvalvular and aortic valvular stenosis murmurs

A subvalvular hypertrophic cardiomyopathic murmur becomes louder during the Valsalva's maneuver, whereas an aortic valvular stenosis murmur doesn't. Performing the Valsalva's maneuver or having the patient stand up suddenly decreases the venous return and left ventricular filling; this makes the left ventricle smaller, the obstruction more severe, and the subvalvular hypertrophic obstructive cardiomyopathic murmur

Auscultatory area for subvalvular aortic stenosis murmur

1. Tricuspid area
2. Mitral area

louder. Having the patient squat increases peripheral vascular resistance and left ventricular filling; this maneuver decreases the pressure gradient across the aortic valve and decreases or obliterates the subvalvular hypertrophic obstructive cardiomyopathic murmur.

SYSTOLIC REGURGITATION MURMURS

An abnormality of either the tricuspid or mitral valve may result in backward turbulent blood flow during systole. This means that blood moves in a direction opposite that of the normal uni-directional flow pattern. Blood regurgitates through a defective, incompetent tricuspid or mitral valve into the left or right atrium, resulting in what is commonly called tricuspid or mitral valve insufficiency. An incompetent valve may be caused by a primary valvular disorder or may develop secondary to dysfunction of the valve's supporting structures.

Regurgitant murmurs heard in patients with these disorders may be early or late systolic or holosystolic. Early systolic murmurs have a crescendo–decrescendo configuration; late systolic murmurs, either a crescendo or crescendo–decrescendo configuration; and holosystolic murmurs, a plateau shape.

Area producing tricuspid regurgitation murmur

Regurgitant tricuspid valve

Tricuspid regurgitation murmurs

A tricuspid regurgitation murmur, also called *tricuspid insufficiency*, most commonly results from right ventricular dilation, which usually results from mitral valve disease or left-sided heart failure but may also be caused by pulmonary disease. It occasionally results from a congenital valve malformation and may also be acquired as a result of infective endocarditis, a right ventricular infarction, or trauma to the valve or its supporting structures.

This murmur can also be heard occasionally in a patient with a transvenous pacemaker because the pacemaker lead interferes with tricuspid valve closure, creating a tricuspid regurgitation-type murmur. The T_1 (tricuspid valve closure) intensity is either increased, normal, or decreased. (◆**Sound 34**)

Sound characteristics

A tricuspid regurgitation murmur is usually heard best over the tricuspid area. In some patients, it's heard only during inspiration. The murmur may radiate to the right of the sternum. Its usual soft intensity may increase during deep inspiration. The murmur's

PCG and ECG showing tricuspid regurgitation murmur

Auscultatory area for tricuspid regurgitation murmur

Tricuspid area

duration is long. It has a medium pitch that's heard best using the diaphragm of the stethoscope and a scratchy or blowing quality. The murmur's timing is systolic: it lasts from S_1 to P_2. On the ECG waveform, the murmur begins just after the QRS complex and ends after the T wave. It is holosystolic and plateau-shaped. (◆Sound 34)

Enhancement techniques
Regardless of a tricuspid regurgitation murmur's cause, the murmur increases in intensity during inspiration because venous return and right ventricular filling are increased, creating higher pressure gradients during systole. To enhance the murmur, have the patient breathe through his mouth slowly, quietly, and more deeply while sitting or standing. Caution the patient not to hold his breath because this negates the maneuver's effect. Another technique is to apply pressure inward and upward below the right costal margin. The murmur is louder during inspiration. In some patients, this is the only time the murmur is audible. The inspiratory increase in the loudness of right-sided auscultatory events is called *Carvallo's sign*.

If a tricuspid regurgitation murmur is secondary to right-sided heart failure, right ventricular filling may be limited with inspiration; consequently, the murmur may not be intensified during deep breathing.

This murmur is rarely accompanied by a systolic thrill, and neither its timing in systole nor its intensity correlates with the severity of the regurgitation.

PCG and ECG showing mitral regurgitation murmur

Area producing mitral regurgitation murmur

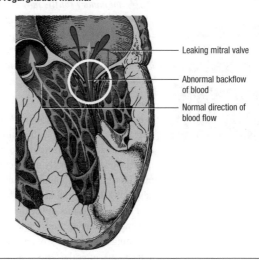

Leaking mitral valve

Abnormal backflow of blood

Normal direction of blood flow

Mitral regurgitation murmurs

A mitral regurgitation murmur, also called *mitral insufficiency*, may be caused by a congenital or acquired abnormality of the mitral valve leaflets, the valve's supporting structures, or the left ventricle. An incompetent mitral valve causes backward blood flow through the incompetent mitral valve during systole. The increased pressure at the aortic valve facilitates regurgitation of blood through the incompetent mitral valve into the low-pressure left atrium, producing a mitral regurgitation murmur. (◆**Sound 35**)

This murmur may appear in early systole, midsystole, or late systole, or it may be holosystolic. Its quality, duration, and radiation depend on the extent, duration, and location of the disease. Usually, late systolic murmurs are associated with mild to moderate regurgitation.

 AGE ISSUE *As a person ages, fibrotic and sclerotic changes thicken the mitral valve leaflets, leading to rigidity and incomplete closure.*

Holosystolic mitral regurgitation murmurs

A holosystolic mitral regurgitation murmur can be caused by the effects of rheumatic heart disease on the mitral valve, by mitral valve prolapse, by left ventricular dilation, or by papillary muscle dysfunction. The murmur can usually be heard regardless of the patient's position, but grade $^1/6$ to $^2/6$ murmurs may be heard best with the patient in the partial left lateral recumbent position or after exercise.

A loud S_3 usually accompanies moderate to severe mitral regurgitation; this sound is related not to heart failure but to the increased left ventricular volume in early diastole.

AGE ISSUE *A systolic or continuous murmur called mammary souffle may be heard in women in the late stages of pregnancy or early in the postpartum period. It's caused by increased breast circulation. Typically, firm pressure to the diaphragm of the stethoscope terminates the murmur. It's heard best with the patient in the supine position on the left or right second or third intercostal spaces.*

Sound characteristics

A holosystolic mitral regurgitation murmur is usually heard best near the heart's apex over the mitral area. The sound may radiate to the axillae or posteriorly over the lung bases. Its intensity is variable and is usually unaffected by respiration; however, it may be somewhat diminished during inspiration. The murmur has a long duration. It has a medium to high pitch that's heard best using the diaphragm of the stethoscope. The murmur may be accompanied by a systolic apical thrill. Its quality is blowing, and its timing is systolic—from S_1 to S_2. On the ECG waveform, it appears just after the QRS complex to the end of the T wave. The murmur is holosystolic and plateau-shaped. (◆**Sound 35**)

Acute mitral regurgitation murmurs

Acute mitral regurgitation is less common than chronic mitral regurgitation. Its murmur results from rupture of the chordae tendineae, papillary muscle, or both. Occasionally, this murmur occurs with a myocardial infarction, but it may also result from severe damage to the mitral valve from trauma or infection.

Auscultatory area for mitral regurgitation murmur

Mitral area

PCG and ECG showing acute mitral regurgitation murmur

ALERT *Rupture of the chordae tendineae may lead to acute pulmonary edema. Notify the physician immediately, and monitor the patient for signs and symptoms of acute pulmonary edema (acute shortage of breath; rapid respiration; audible wheezes and crackles; productive cough that produces frothy, blood-tinged sputum; tachycardia; hypotension; and cyanotic, cold, clammy skin).*

An acute mitral regurgitation murmur begins with mitral valve closure and has a decrescendo configuration. (◆**Sound 36**) Its intensity decreases as ventricular and atrial pressures equilibrate during late systole. An S_4 is usually heard with acute mitral regurgitation.

Sound characteristics

An acute mitral regurgitation murmur is usually heard best near the heart's apex over the mitral area. Its intensity is usually loud (grade 4/6 to 6/6 if the murmur results from rupture of the chordae tendineae). It's accompanied by a systolic thrill. The murmur's duration is medium long. It has a high pitch that's heard best using the diaphragm of the stethoscope and a quality that can be musical. Its timing is systolic: it begins with M_1 and ends with or before A_2. On the ECG waveform, the murmur begins just after the QRS complex and ends just after the T wave. In many patients, it is holosystolic and wedge-shaped (the wedge shape has a steeper decrescendo configuration). (◆**Sound 36**)

Area producing mitral valve prolapse murmur

1. Enlarged leaflets
2. Normal mitral valve position

PCG and ECG showing mitral valve prolapse murmur

Mitral valve prolapse murmurs

The murmur associated with a prolapsed mitral valve usually appears in late systole and is either isolated or accompanied by a nonejection midsystolic click or clicks caused by the mitral valve prolapsing and ballooning up into the left atrium. This is sometimes referred to as the click murmur syndrome. (◆Sound 37)

 AGE ISSUE *Mitral valve prolapse is one of the most common valvular abnormalities found in adults.*

Sound characteristics

A mitral valve prolapse murmur is usually heard best near the heart's apex over the mitral area. Its intensity is usually soft (grade $2/6$ to $3/6$), and its duration is short. It has a high pitch that's heard best using the diaphragm of the stethoscope. The murmur has a musical quality; when loud, it's sometimes described as a whoop or honk. Although its timing is usually late systolic, it can sometimes be holosystolic. On the ECG waveform, the murmur coincides with the T wave and ends just after the T wave. It has a crescendo or crescendo–decrescendo configuration. (◆Sound 37)

Enhancement techniques

Having the patient stand decreases the left ventricular volume, which causes the mitral valve prolapse murmur to be heard earlier in systole, to be louder, and to last longer. Having the patient squat increases the left ventricular volume, which causes the murmur to be heard later in systole.

Auscultatory area for mitral valve prolapse murmur

Mitral area

PCG and ECG showing a ventricular septal defect murmur

The direction in which a mitral valve prolapse murmur is transmitted across the chest wall depends on the disease. For example, if the mitral valve's posterior leaflet is involved, blood flow might be directed more anteriorly and medially. Consequently, the murmur would be transmitted toward the heart's base and heard best over the aortic area and along the left sternal edge. If the anterior leaflet is incompetent, blood flow is directed posteriorly against the posterior left atrial wall, and the murmur is transmitted toward the left axilla and back.

VENTRICULAR SEPTAL DEFECT MURMUR

A ventricular septal defect (VSD) is an opening—usually in the membranous portion of the ventricular septum—that allows direct communication between the ventricles. Typically, blood shunts from left to right because of higher pressures in the left ventricle.

AGE ISSUE *Murmurs in pediatric patients are typically associated with ventricular septal defects, patent ductus arteriosus, atrial septal defects, and mitral valve prolapse.*

Sound characteristics

A VSD murmur is heard over the lower sternal border and, if loud, can be heard over the entire precordium. A thrill may be palpable along the lower left sternal border. The murmur is holosystolic. S_2 is widely split because the aortic valve closes early. If the VSD is large, pulmonary hypertension eventually

Area producing ventricular septal defect murmur

Ventricular septal defect

Auscultatory area for ventricular septal defect murmur

1. Precordial area
2. Left sternal border

develops, the S_2 narrows, and the P_2 becomes louder than the A_2. The intensity and pitch vary with the size of the VSD. If pulmonary hypertension becomes severe, shunting may stop and the P_2 and A_2 may merge.

◀◀◀ POSTTEST

1. Describe the characteristics of an SEM.
2. Describe the characteristics of a supravalvular pulmonic stenosis murmur.
3. Describe the characteristics of a pulmonic valvular stenosis murmur.
4. Describe the characteristics of a subvalvular pulmonic stenosis murmur.
5. Describe the characteristics of a supravalvular aortic stenosis murmur.
6. Describe the characteristics of an aortic valvular stenosis murmur.
7. Describe the characteristics of a subvalvular aortic stenosis murmur.
8. Describe the characteristics of a tricuspid regurgitation murmur.
9. Describe the characteristics of a holosystolic mitral regurgitation murmur.
10. Describe the characteristics of an acute mitral regurgitation murmur.
11. Describe the characteristics of a mitral valve prolapse murmur.

Diastolic murmurs

CHAPTER 9

PRETEST ►►►

1. How is the sound of a diastolic murmur produced?
2. List the aortic regurgitation murmurs.
3. List the pulmonic regurgitation murmurs.
4. What are the characteristics of a mitral stenosis murmur?
5. What are the characteristics of a tricuspid stenosis murmur?

ANATOMY AND PHYSIOLOGY

At the end of ventricular systole and the beginning of diastole, the aortic and pulmonic valves close. During this time, the A_2-P_2 interval can usually be auscultated. After a brief period of isovolumic relaxation, the mitral and tricuspid valves open, and blood flows from the atria into the ventricles. During this early filling period, a third heart sound (S_3)—which sounds like "Ken-Tuc-Key"—can sometimes be heard in healthy individuals younger than age 20. Late in diastole, the atria contract, increasing blood flow into the ventricles. Occasionally, a fourth heart sound can be heard during this late filling period. Except for these brief heart sounds, diastole is normally silent. When diastolic murmurs occur, they are heard between the second and first heart sounds (S_2 and S_1) or between the end of the T wave and the beginning of the QRS complex on the electrocardiogram (ECG) waveform.

The regurgitation of blood through the aortic and pulmonic valves may cause diastolic murmurs. Because both valves close at the beginning of diastole, murmurs produced by dysfunctional aortic and pulmonic valves begin early in diastole, immediately after the affected valve closes.

Mitral and tricuspid valve stenosis and conditions that produce turbulent blood flow across normal mitral or tricuspid valves also cause diastolic murmurs. Because these valves open after a period of isovolumic relaxation, these murmurs are heard during mid-diastole.

AORTIC REGURGITATION MURMURS

Early diastolic aortic regurgitation murmurs

The early diastolic aortic regurgitation murmur, also called *aortic insufficiency*, can result from rheumatic heart disease, Marfan syndrome, osteogenesis imperfecta, a congenital bicuspid valve, or

PCG and ECG showing early diastolic aortic regurgitation murmur

Area producing early diastolic aortic regurgitation murmur

Regurgitant aortic valve

Auscultatory area for early diastolic aortic regurgitation murmur

1. Aortic area
2. Pulmonic area
3. Erb's point
4. Mitral area

a dissecting aortic aneurysm. Leakage around a prosthetic aortic valve can also produce this murmur.

Because the aortic pressure normally exceeds the left ventricular pressure at the beginning of diastole, it forces a retrograde, or backward, flow of blood across an incompetent aortic valve. The turbulent blood flow produces the murmur. In this murmur, A_2 may sound normal, or it may be accentuated if the patient has severe systemic hypertension. (◆**Sound 38**) This murmur is commonly associated with a systolic ejection murmur produced by increased left ventricular stroke volume.

Sound characteristics
The early diastolic aortic regurgitation murmur is usually heard best near the heart's base over the aortic and pulmonic areas, over Erb's point, and near the heart's apex over the mitral area. Because of its usually soft intensity, it's heard best in a quiet environment. The murmur can last throughout most of diastole. It has a high pitch that's heard best using the diaphragm of the stethoscope, and it has a blowing or musical quality. Its timing is diastolic, beginning with A_2. On the ECG waveform, the murmur begins after the T wave and ends just before the QRS complex. It has a decrescendo configuration. (◆**Sound 38**)

If aortic regurgitation is associated with aortic root dilation or with a dissecting aneurysm of the ascending aorta, the diastolic murmur may be louder along the right sternal border between the second and fourth intercostal spaces than along the left sternal border between the second and fourth intercostal spaces, respectively. If the patient is elderly or has chronic obstructive pulmonary disease, the murmur may be heard best near the heart's

PCG and ECG showing middiastolic aortic regurgitation (Austin Flint) murmur

apex over the mitral area. If the murmur is loud, it may be heard over most of the precordium.

Enhancement techniques

This murmur can be enhanced by having the patient sit down, lean forward, and hold his breath after expiration or perform maneuvers that increase aortic diastolic pressure, such as squatting or performing the handgrip exercise.

Middiastolic aortic regurgitation (Austin Flint) murmurs

Severe aortic regurgitation may be associated with a middiastolic and presystolic rumbling murmur. This murmur is caused by the aortic regurgitant jet impinging on the normal mitral inflow and augmenting mitral inflow turbulence. The murmur generated by the turbulent blood flow across the mitral valve is called an *Austin Flint murmur*; it may be confused with a murmur of mitral stenosis. (◆**Sound 39**)

Sound characteristics

The Austin Flint murmur is usually heard best near the heart's apex over the mitral area. It's introduced with an S_3 rather than an opening snap (OS), as occurs in mitral stenosis. Its intensity is usually soft. It has a low pitch that's heard best using the bell of the stethoscope. The murmur has a rumbling quality. Its timing is confined to middiastole or presystolic. It's heard just before the QRS complex on the ECG waveform. The murmur has a presystolic crescendo configuration; its middiastolic component has a crescendo–decrescendo configuration. (◆**Sound 39**)

Area producing middiastolic aortic regurgitation (Austin Flint) murmur

1. Regurgitant aortic valve
2. Anterior mitral leaflet

Auscultatory area for middiastolic aortic regurgitation (Austin Flint) murmur

Mitral area

PCG and ECG showing Graham Steell murmur

Area producing Graham Steell murmur

1. Dilated pulmonary artery
2. Regurgitant pulmonic valve

Auscultatory area for Graham Steell murmur

1. Third intercostal space
2. Fourth intercostal space

PULMONIC REGURGITATION MURMURS

Graham Steell murmurs

Because the pulmonary artery pressure is normally quite low during diastole, significant regurgitation from a normal pulmonic valve rarely occurs without pulmonary hypertension. Pulmonary hypertension produces pulmonary artery dilation and a relative pulmonic insufficiency because of dilation of the pulmonic valve ring. (◆Sound 40) A pulmonic regurgitation murmur resulting from pulmonary hypertension is called a *Graham Steell murmur.*

Sound characteristics

A Graham Steell murmur secondary to pulmonary hypertension is usually heard best along the left sternal border over the third and fourth intercostal spaces. It isn't transmitted to the right sternum. Its intensity is usually loud and its duration variable. The murmur has a high pitch that's heard best using the diaphragm of the stethoscope, and it has a blowing quality. Its timing is early diastolic, beginning with a loud P_2. Sometimes an ejection sound can be heard. The murmur is heard after the end of the T wave on the ECG waveform and usually doesn't extend to S_1. It has a decrescendo configuration. (◆Sound 40)

Enhancement techniques

The Graham Steell murmur is intensified during inspiration.

Normal pressure pulmonic valve murmurs

When a murmur results from idiopathic pulmonary artery dilation or congenital pulmonary valve insufficiency, the pulmonary artery

PCG and ECG showing normal pressure pulmonic valve murmur

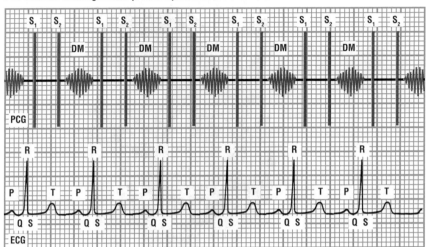

diastolic pressure isn't elevated. Regurgitation is delayed until the right ventricular pressure has fallen below the pulmonary artery diastolic pressure during isovolumic relaxation. (◆**Sound 41**)

Sound characteristics
The normal pressure pulmonic valve murmur is usually heard best along the left sternal border over the third and fourth intercostal spaces. It isn't transmitted to the right sternum. Its intensity is soft and its duration brief. The murmur has a low pitch that's heard best using the bell of the stethoscope. It has a rumbling quality, and its timing is early to middiastolic. It begins shortly after P_2 is heard. In the ECG waveform, it begins after the T wave and ends before the P wave. The murmur has a crescendo–decrescendo configuration. (◆**Sound 41**)

Enhancement techniques
The normal pressure pulmonic valve murmur is intensified during inspiration.

OTHER DIASTOLIC MURMURS

Mitral stenosis murmurs
Mitral stenosis results from a congenital defect or chronic rheumatic valvulitis. Typically, valvulitis results in scarring and calcification of the valve, causing it to cease normal function. The scarring and calcification create a funnel-shaped opening between the left atrium and left ventricle.

A mitral stenosis murmur starts with an OS after A_2 and isovolumic relaxation (◆**Sound 42**); this OS is an important

Area producing normal pressure pulmonic valve murmur

1. Dilated pulmonary artery
2. Regurgitant pulmonic valve

Auscultatory area for normal pressure pulmonic valve murmur

1. Third intercostal space
2. Fourth intercostal space

Area producing mitral stenosis murmur

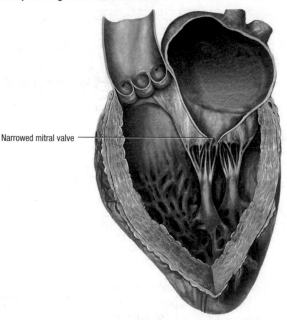

Narrowed mitral valve

Auscultatory area for mitral stenosis murmur

Mitral area

diagnostic feature of mitral stenosis. The murmur is produced by rapid, turbulent blood flow through a rigid, narrowed mitral valve opening. Turbulence increases just before systole; this gives the murmur its characteristic presystolic crescendo.

The more severe the stenosis, the longer the duration of the murmur. With severe mitral stenosis, the murmur is holodiastolic; in moderate stenosis, it appears in early and late diastole. The murmur ends with a loud M_1, which implies that the valve leaflets are mobile; the M_1 is usually palpable. If the valve is calcified, S_1 is soft and an OS isn't heard.

Mitral stenosis is sometimes associated with mitral regurgitation, so a systolic murmur may be heard as well. If mitral stenosis has caused pulmonary hypertension and right-sided heart failure, tricuspid regurgitation may be the dominant murmur heard.

Sound characteristics

A mitral stenosis murmur is usually heard best near the heart's apex over the mitral area. Its intensity and duration vary. It has a low pitch that's heard best using the bell of the stethoscope and a rumbling quality that has been compared to thunder. The timing of a mitral stenosis murmur is diastolic: it begins after A_2 with an OS and ends with a loud M_1. (◆**Sound 42**) However, stenosis severity affects the duration of the murmur.

PCG and ECG showing mitral stenosis murmur (atrial fibrillation)

PCG and ECG showing mitral stenosis murmur (normal sinus rhythm)

On the ECG waveform, the murmur begins just after the T wave and ends during the QRS complex. It has a crescendo–decrescendo configuration. In patients with a normal sinus rhythm, the presystolic component has a crescendo configuration. (◆**Sound 43)** (See *PCG and ECG showing mitral stenosis murmur [atrial fibrillation]* and *PCG and ECG showing mitral stenosis murmur [normal sinus rhythm].*)

PCG and ECG showing tricuspid stenosis murmur

Area producing tricuspid stenosis murmur

Stenotic tricuspid valve

Auscultatory area for tricuspid stenosis murmur

Tricuspid area

Enhancement techniques

The mitral stenosis murmur is heard best with the patient in a partial left lateral recumbent position. It can be intensified by maneuvers that increase the cardiac output, such as having the patient exercise for a few minutes, raise his legs from a recumbent position, or cough several times.

Tricuspid stenosis murmurs

Tricuspid stenosis rarely occurs as an isolated defect; it's almost always associated with mitral valve defects. A tricuspid stenosis murmur begins shortly after a normal S_2 and is introduced by an OS that can be seen on a phonocardiogram (PCG) but that is seldom heard. (◆**Sound 44**)

Sound characteristics

A tricuspid stenosis murmur is usually heard best over the tricuspid area. Its usually soft intensity increases during inspiration and fades or disappears during expiration.

The duration of the murmur varies. It has a low pitch that's heard best using the bell of the stethoscope while the patient is in the partial left lateral recumbent position. The murmur has a rumbling quality. Its timing is mid- to late diastolic: it ends just before S_1. An OS may be heard. On the ECG waveform, the murmur begins just after the T wave and ends just before the QRS complex. In patients with a normal sinus rhythm, it has a late diastolic crescendo or crescendo–decrescendo configuration. (◆**Sound 44**)

AUSCULTATION TIP *The tricuspid stenosis murmur can be differentiated from the mitral stenosis murmur because the murmur intensifies with inspiration, whereas the mitral stenosis murmur doesn't.*

◀◀◀ POSTTEST

1. Describe the characteristics of an early diastolic aortic regurgitation murmur.
2. How can an early diastolic aortic regurgitation murmur be enhanced?
3. Describe the characteristics of an Austin Flint murmur.
4. Describe the characteristics of a Graham Steell murmur.
5. Describe the characteristics of a normal pressure pulmonic valve murmur.
6. How is a normal pressure pulmonic valve murmur enhanced?
7. How is the sound of a mitral stenosis murmur produced?
8. Describe the characteristics of a mitral stenosis murmur.
9. How is a mitral stenosis murmur enhanced?
10. Describe the characteristics of a tricuspid stenosis murmur.

10 Continuous murmurs

1. How is the sound of a continuous murmur produced?
2. What is a cervical venous hum?
3. Why do the sounds of a patent ductus arteriosus (PDA) murmur change with age?
4. How can you differentiate between a PDA murmur and cervical venous hum murmur?

TWO CAUSES

Continuous murmurs are generated by rapid blood flow through arteries or veins or by shunting. Shunting occurs when an abnormal communication is created between the high-pressure arterial system and the low-pressure venous system. The murmurs begin in systole and persist, without interruption, through the second heart sound (S_2) into diastole. Because these murmurs end late in diastole, they are continuous throughout the cardiac cycle.

CERVICAL VENOUS HUM MURMURS

The most common continuous murmur is a normal cervical venous hum, caused by rapid downward blood flow through the jugular veins in the lower part of the neck. (◆Sound 45) A cervical venous hum is present in most individuals, but it's more pronounced in patients with hyperkinetic circulatory states, such as anemia, pregnancy, and thyrotoxicosis. The hum will disappear if the patient performs the Valsalva's maneuver, lies down, or has pressure applied over the jugular vein.

Sound characteristics
A cervical venous hum murmur is heard best over the right supraclavicular fossa when the patient is sitting and his head is turned to the left. It has a faint intensity that increases during diastole. The murmur has a long duration: it lasts throughout the cardiac

PCG and ECG showing cervical venous murmur

cycle. Its high pitch is heard best using the diaphragm of the stethoscope. Its quality is soft and its timing continuous. The hum is louder between S_2 and the first heart sound (S_1). (◆**Sound 45**) The murmur has a plateau shape in systole and a crescendo–decrescendo configuration in diastole.

PATENT DUCTUS ARTERIOSUS MURMURS

A PDA murmur is the prototype of continuous murmurs. (◆**Sound 46**) Normally, the ductus is open during fetal life and closes shortly after birth. When the ductus remains open, abnormal blood flow, or shunting, occurs from the high-pressure aorta to the low-pressure pulmonary artery. The PDA murmur extends into diastole. A thrill may be palpable with a loud PDA murmur.

Sound characteristics

A PDA murmur is heard best over the entire left first and second intercostal spaces. Its intensity is faint when the murmur is limited to this area. If the murmur is loud, the systolic component may be heard along the left sternal border or over the mitral area. A loud PDA murmur may radiate to the back between the

Auscultatory area for cervical venous hum murmur

Supraclavicular fossa

PCG and ECG showing patent ductus arteriosus murmur

Area producing patent ductus arteriosus murmur

1. Aorta
2. PDA
3. Pulmonary artery

Auscultatory area for patent ductus arteriosus murmur

1. First intercostal space
2. Second intercostal space
3. Left sternal border
4. Mitral area

scapulae. A PDA murmur has a long duration. Its intensity varies, roughly correlating with the ductus size; typically, the murmur reaches maximum intensity late in systole and then fades during diastole.

A PDA murmur has a high pitch heard equally well using the bell or diaphragm of the stethoscope. It has a rough, machinery-like quality, and its timing is continuous. It begins with—or shortly after—a normal S_1 and disappears just before the next S_1. Because the murmur peaks in late systole, S_2 may be difficult to hear. S_2 may be paradoxically split if the left ventricular ejection time is prolonged. A third heart sound may be heard over the mitral area. (◆**Sound 46**) The murmur has a crescendo–decrescendo configuration.

Enhancement techniques
Exercise can increase the intensity and duration of a PDA murmur.

Differentiating PDA murmurs from cervical venous hum murmurs

To differentiate these PDA murmurs from cervical venous hum murmurs, remember that the hum is loudest above the clavicle, is usually heard better on the right, and can be obliterated by pressing on the jugular vein or placing the patient in a supine position. A venous hum is truly continuous and is usually louder during diastole.

◀◀◀POSTTEST

1. How is the sound of a continuous murmur produced?
2. What causes a cervical venous hum?
3. Describe the characteristics of a cervical venous hum murmur.
4. Describe the characteristics of a PDA murmur.
5. How can a PDA murmur be enhanced?
6. How can you differentiate between a PDA murmur and a cervical venous hum murmur?

Other auscultatory sounds

PRETEST ◆◆◆

1. What are the four types of prosthetic valves?
2. What are the similarities and differences of the sounds produced by the four types of aortic prosthetic valves?
3. What are the similarities and differences of the sounds produced by the four types of mitral prosthetic valves?
4. What produces a pericardial friction rub?
5. What is mediastinal crunch?

PROSTHETIC VALVE SOUNDS AND MURMURS

Prosthetic heart valves—such as the ball-in-cage, tilting-disk, bileaflet, and porcine valves—are used to replace malfunctioning human valves. The aortic and mitral valves are the ones most commonly replaced. The tricuspid valve is replaced occasionally; the pulmonic valve, rarely. The following discussion focuses on the aortic and mitral valves.

AGE ISSUE *Because mechanical valves last a long time, they're usually inserted in children and adults younger than age 40. However, these valves shouldn't be inserted in women of childbearing age because mechanical valve implantation requires the patient to take an oral anticoagulant, such as warfarin, which can cause birth defects if taken during the first trimester of pregnancy.*

General characteristics

When a prosthetic valve is surgically placed in the aortic orifice, it's positioned so that it opens during systole and closes at the beginning of diastole. However, when a prosthetic valve is surgically placed in the mitral orifice, it's positioned so that it closes at the beginning of systole and opens during diastole.

An aortic prosthetic valve won't change a normal first heart sound (S₁), and a mitral prosthetic valve will not change a

Auscultatory area for aortic and mitral prosthetic valve murmurs with systolic ejection murmur

1. Aortic area
2. Tricuspid area
3. Mitral area

normal second heart sound (S$_2$). However, prosthetic valves do produce characteristic auscultatory sounds and murmurs. For example, some prostheses produce opening clicks, and all prostheses, regardless of type or position, produce closing clicks. The ball-in-cage valve produces the loudest sounds.

Typically, any disappearance or muffling of previously heard prosthetic valve sounds or murmurs, or the development of a new murmur in a patient with a prosthetic valve, indicates possible prosthetic valve dysfunction.

Almost all prosthetic valves in the aortic position are associated with a soft early systolic or midsystolic ejection murmur. This murmur is heard best over the tricuspid, mitral, and aortic areas and is similar to the mild aortic stenosis murmur.

Some prosthetic valves in the mitral position produce a short, soft, rumbling early diastolic murmur, which is very similar to the mitral stenosis murmur except that it's brief and a presystolic component isn't heard. This murmur is heard best near the heart's apex over the mitral area while the patient is in the partial left lateral recumbent position.

Auscultatory area for mitral prosthetic valve murmur with early diastolic murmur

Mitral area

AORTIC PROSTHETIC VALVES

Distinctive sounds and murmurs are associated with the various types of prostheses used in aortic valve replacement. (◆Sound 47)

Aortic ball-in-cage valve
A normally functioning aortic ball-in-cage valve prosthesis doesn't change the normal S$_1$ characteristics. S$_1$ is followed by an aortic opening click that's louder than S$_1$; it's sharp and high-pitched, and it has a crisp quality. An aortic closing click replaces A$_2$. Although the aortic ball-in-cage valve prosthesis is no longer inserted, patients with this type of prosthesis may still be seen.

PCG showing aortic ball-in-cage valve murmur

PCG

S_1

SM

P_2

Valve opens

Valve closes

Sound characteristics

The murmur generated by an aortic ball-in-cage valve prosthesis is usually heard best near the apex over the mitral and aortic areas and along the left sternal border. Its intensity is usually loud and easy to hear, and its duration variable. It has a medium pitch that's heard best using the diaphragm of the stethoscope. The murmur has a crunchy, harsh quality. Its timing is midsystolic. The interval between the aortic closing click and P_2 is similar to the normal A_2-P_2 interval, and it normally widens during inspiration. The murmur has a crescendo–decrescendo configuration.

Detecting a malfunctioning aortic ball-in-cage valve

Dysfunction of an aortic ball-in-cage valve prosthesis commonly causes the aortic opening click to become soft or absent; the aortic closing click may also be absent. A diastolic murmur and a long systolic ejection murmur (SEM) may appear.

Aortic tilting-disk valve

S_1 is unchanged with abnormally functioning aortic tilting-disk valve prosthesis. An aortic opening click may be heard, and the interval between the aortic closing click and P_2 is normal. The aortic closing click isn't as loud as the click heard with a ball-in-cage prosthesis.

Sound characteristics

The murmur generated by an aortic tilting-disk valve prosthesis is usually heard best near the apex over the mitral and aortic areas and along the left sternal border. Its intensity is usually soft (grade) and its duration short. It has a medium pitch heard best with the diaphragm of the stethoscope. The murmur has a rough or harsh quality. Its timing is systolic. The interval between the aortic closing click and P_2 is similar to the normal A_2-P_2 interval, and it widens during inspiration. The murmur has a crescendo–decrescendo configuration.

PCG showing aortic tilting disk valve murmur

PCG

S_1

SM

Valve opens   Valve closes

Dotted line indicates that valve opening may or may not be heard.

Tilting-disk valve

PCG showing aortic bileaflet valve murmur

PCG

S_1

SM

Valve opens   Valve closes

Bileaflet valve

Detecting a malfunctioning aortic tilting-disk valve

Dysfunction of an aortic tilting-disk valve prosthesis commonly causes some or all of the following changes: the aortic closing click may be absent, a diastolic murmur may be heard, or a longer SEM may appear.

Aortic bileaflet valve

S_1 is normal with a normally functioning aortic bileaflet valve prosthesis. The aortic opening click is commonly inaudible, but the closing click is loud and distinct.

Sound characteristics

The murmur generated by an aortic bileaflet valve prosthesis is usually heard best near the apex over the mitral and aortic areas and along the left sternal border with the patient in the left lateral position. Its intensity is usually soft (grade $2/6$) and its duration short. It has a medium pitch that's heard best using the diaphragm of the stethoscope. The murmur has a rough or harsh quality, and its timing is systolic. The interval between the aortic closing click and P_2 is similar to the normal A_2-P_2 interval, and it widens during inspiration. The murmur has a crescendo–decrescendo configuration.

Porcine valve

Carpentier–Edwards Duraflex tissue valve. Used with permission of Edwards Lifesciences Corporation.

PCG showing aortic porcine valve murmur

Detecting a malfunctioning aortic bileaflet valve

Dysfunction of the aortic bileaflet valve prosthesis may cause the aortic closing click to disappear, a diastolic murmur to appear, or both. A longer SEM also may appear.

Aortic porcine valve

S_2 is normal with a properly functioning aortic porcine valve prosthesis. There's no opening click in a properly functioning porcine valve.

> **AGE ISSUE** *Porcine valves are better suited for older patients because in younger patients, especially those younger than age 40, they're prone to calcification. Furthermore, porcine valves gradually deteriorate and must be replaced, making them less desirable for a patient who wants to avoid future surgery. However, because these valves don't require anticoagulation therapy, they may be an option for women who are pregnant or of childbearing age.*

Sound characteristics

The murmur generated by an aortic porcine valve prosthesis is usually heard best near the apex over the mitral and aortic areas and along the left sternal border. Its intensity is usually soft (grade $2/6$) and its duration short. It has a medium pitch that's heard best using the diaphragm of the stethoscope. The murmur has a rough or harsh quality, and its timing is systolic.

The interval between the aortic closing sound and P_2 is similar to the normal A_2-P_2 interval, and it widens during inspiration. The murmur has a crescendo–decrescendo configuration.

PCG showing mitral ball-in-cage valve sounds

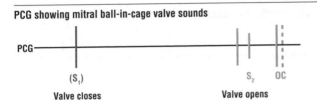

Parentheses around S_1 indicate that S_1 will not be heard because valve closure is louder. Dotted line indicates that opening click (OC) may or may not be heard.

Detecting a malfunctioning aortic porcine valve
Dysfunction of an aortic porcine valve prosthesis may cause a diastolic murmur to appear. A longer SEM also may appear.

MITRAL PROSTHETIC VALVES

Distinctive sounds and murmurs are associated with the various types of prostheses used in mitral valve replacement.
(◆Sound 48)

Mitral ball-in-cage valve
The mitral closing click replaces M_1 with a normally functioning mitral ball-in-cage valve prosthesis. Patients with this type of prosthetic valve have an opening click after S_2 and may have middiastolic clicks or short, soft (grade 2/6), rumbling diastolic murmurs that are heard best near the apex over the mitral area with the patient in a partial left lateral recumbent position.

Sound characteristics
M_1 is loud and higher in frequency. A mitral opening click follows a normal S_2.

Detecting a malfunctioning mitral ball-in-cage valve
Dysfunction of a mitral ball-in-cage valve prosthesis may cause some or all of the following changes: the sounds normally associated with the valve may vary in intensity in a patient with normal sinus rhythm; a short interval between A_2 and the mitral opening click may occur, indicating high left atrial pressure; a holosystolic murmur may occur, indicating mitral regurgitation; or the intensity and duration of the diastolic murmur may change, indicating mitral obstruction.

PCG showing mitral tilting-disk valve sounds

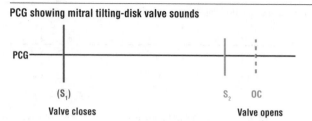

Parentheses around S₁ indicate that S₁ will not be heard because valve closure is louder. Dotted line indicates that opening click (OC) may or may not be heard.

Mitral tilting-disk valve

A normally functioning mitral tilting-disk valve prosthesis replaces M_1 with a mitral closing click. This closing click is always distinctly audible and high-pitched; its maximum intensity is located near the apex over the mitral area.

Sound characteristics

A mitral opening click may follow a normal S_2.

Detecting a malfunctioning mitral tilting-disk valve

Dysfunction of a mitral tilting-disk valve prosthesis may cause some or all of the following changes: the mitral closing click may be absent, a new diastolic murmur may develop, a previously auscultated diastolic murmur may intensify, or a holosystolic mitral regurgitation murmur may appear.

Mitral bileaflet valve

A normally functioning mitral bileaflet valve prosthesis replaces M_1 with a mitral closing click that's loud and high-pitched. The mitral opening click, however, may be inaudible. If it is audible, it follows a normal S_2. In some patients with a mitral bileaflet valve prosthesis, a short middiastolic rumble occurs; this rumble is heard best near the apex over the mitral area.

Sound characteristics

The first sound is replaced by a higher-pitched sound. The mitral opening click, though rarely heard, follows a normal S_2.

Detecting a malfunctioning mitral bileaflet valve

Dysfunction of a mitral bileaflet valve prosthesis may cause a holosystolic murmur, a new diastolic murmur, or both to appear.

PCG showing mitral bileaflet valve sounds

Parentheses around S$_1$ indicate that S$_1$ will not be heard because valve closure is louder. Dotted line indicates that opening click (OC) may or may not be heard.

PCG showing mitral porcine valve sounds

Parentheses around S$_1$ indicate that S$_1$ will not be heard because valve closure is louder.

Mitral porcine valve

A normally functioning mitral porcine valve prosthesis generates a mitral closing sound that's heard over the mitral area and sounds like a normal M$_1$. No opening sound is heard with this type of valve.

Sound characteristics

This sound is heard best near the apex over the mitral area.

Detecting a malfunctioning mitral porcine valve

Dysfunction of a mitral porcine valve prosthesis may cause a holosystolic mitral regurgitation murmur, a diastolic rumble associated with mitral stenosis, or both to appear.

Auscultatory area for pericardial friction rub

1. Tricuspid area
2. Xyphoid area

PERICARDIAL FRICTION RUBS

When inflamed pericardial surfaces rub together, they produce characteristic high-pitched friction noises known as *pericardial friction rubs*. (◆**Sound 48)** These rubs are a classic sign of pericarditis (inflammation of the pericardium, the sac surrounding the heart), which can be caused by viral or bacterial infections, radiation therapy to the chest, or cardiac trauma. Pericardial friction rubs may also be heard after a pericardiotomy and for a few hours to a few days after a myocardial infarction.

Sound characteristics

A pericardial friction rub is usually heard best, and is sometimes palpable, over the tricuspid and xiphoid areas. It's usually loud and may get louder during inspiration. The rub has a high pitch heard best with the diaphragm of the stethoscope, and it has a grating or scratchy quality. It's usually heard during each cardiac cycle. It has a systolic component and an early and late diastolic component. (◆**Sound 49)** The diastolic components may last for only a few hours.

 AUSCULTATION TIP *To differentiate a pericardial friction rub from a pleural friction rub, have the patient hold his breath. When he does so, a pericardial friction rub will persist, but a pleural friction rub will become inaudible.*

MEDIASTINAL CRUNCH

Heart movements can displace air that's present in the mediastinum; this displacement produces crunchy noises, known as *mediastinal crunch*, which may occur randomly or in a consistent pattern. (◆**Sound 50)** Patients with mediastinal crunch commonly have subcutaneous emphysema (air trapped beneath the skin). You can assess for this condition by palpating for crepitation in the neck.

Sound characteristics

The noises produced by mediastinal crunch are usually heard best along the left sternal border with the patient in a sitting position. The noises have a crunching quality, which may become louder during inspiration. (◆**Sound 50**)

Auscultatory area for mediastinal crunch

1. Left sternal border
2. Mitral area

◀◀◀ POSTTEST

1. Describe the characteristics of an aortic ball-in-cage valve murmur.
2. Describe the characteristics of an aortic tilting-disk murmur.
3. Describe the characteristics of an aortic bileaflet valve murmur.
4. Describe the characteristics of an aortic porcine valve murmur.
5. Describe the characteristics of a mitral ball-in-cage valve murmur.
6. Describe the characteristics of a mitral tilting-disk murmur.
7. Describe the characteristics of a mitral bileaflet valve murmur.
8. Describe the characteristics of a mitral porcine valve murmur.
9. Describe the characteristics of a pericardial friction rub.
10. Describe the characteristics of mediastinal crunch.

Breath sound fundamentals

12 The respiratory system and auscultation

PRETEST ▶▶▶

1. What is the primary function of the respiratory system?
2. Where are the apex and base of the lung located?
3. Describe the process of normal breathing.
4. Which three chest wall surfaces are included in breath sound auscultation?
5. What is the auscultatory sequence?

ANATOMY AND PHYSIOLOGY

The primary function of the respiratory system is the exchange of oxygen (O_2) and carbon dioxide (CO_2) between the alveoli and the pulmonary circulation.

During inspiration, air enters the upper airway and travels through the lower airways until it reaches the alveoli. Each alveolus is surrounded by multiple capillaries. During systole, deoxygenated blood returning from the body's cells is pumped from the right ventricle through the arterial pulmonary circulation to the alveolar capillaries. CO_2 diffuses from the capillary blood across the alveolar capillary membrane and enters the alveolar air. Simultaneously, O_2 from the inspired atmospheric air in the alveolus crosses the alveolar capillary membrane and enters the pulmonary capillary blood.

During expiration, CO_2 is exhaled from the lungs. Oxygenated capillary blood travels to the left side of the heart and is pumped from the ventricle into arterial circulation to the cells of the body, where cellular respiration occurs.

Upper airway

The upper airway consists of the nasal cavities and the pharynx. Air enters the body through the nostrils and passes through the nasal cavities. Vibrissae located in the nostrils filter out foreign

CO_2-O_2 exchange in the alveoli

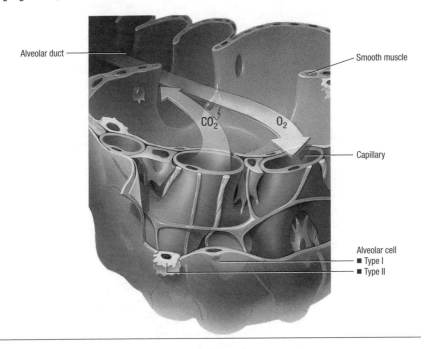

Alveolar duct

Smooth muscle

CO_2

O_2

Capillary

Alveolar cell
- Type I
- Type II

---

particles. The lateral walls of the nasal cavities curve, forming turbinates (conchae), which increase the mucosal surface area and produce turbulent airflow.

The lining of the nasal cavities contains a dense capillary network and serous glands that warm and humidify the inspired air. Seromucous glands produce a sticky film over the lining that traps particles against it during airflow.

The pharynx is divided into three sections: the nasopharynx, the oropharynx, and the hypopharynx. The nasopharynx begins at the posterior openings of the nasal cavities and extends to the soft palate; the oropharynx, the middle section, is the common passageway for food and air; and the hypopharynx, the lower section, extends from the roof of the tongue to the glottic area.

AGE ISSUE *In children, the larynx and glottis are positioned higher in the neck, creating a greater risk for aspiration.*

Location of nasal cavity and pharynx

1
2

1. Nasal cavity
2. Pharynx

Location of turbinates and airflow pattern in the nasal cavity

1
2

1. Turbinates
2. Airflow

Location of nasopharynx, oropharynx, and hypopharynx

Nasopharynx

Oropharynx

Hypopharynx

Lower airway

The lower airway is called the *tracheobronchial tree*. It begins at the level of the cricoid cartilage of the larynx and ends at the distal bronchioles, which open into the alveoli.

The larynx, which contains the epiglottis and vocal cords, has a role in ventilation and phonation and helps protect the lower airway from aspiration.

Trachea

The adult trachea is about 1″ (2.5 cm) in diameter and 4″ (10 cm) long to the bifurcation, which is also called the *carina*. Anteriorly, the trachea begins just below the larynx and is located within the thoracic cavity, beneath the upper two-thirds of the sternum. Posteriorly, it begins at the level of the sixth cervical or first thoracic vertebra and extends to about the fifth thoracic vertebra.

 AGE ISSUE *In children, the trachea is shorter with a more acute angle at the bifurcation of the right bronchus. The smaller diameter of the trachea results in increased airway resistance.*

Mainstem bronchus

The trachea divides into a right and left mainstem bronchus. The left mainstem bronchus leaves the trachea at a sharper angle than the right mainstem bronchus and passes under the aortic arch before entering the lung. The mainstem bronchi enter the lungs at the hila, where the lung tissue attaches to the mediastinum. The bronchi course downward and immediately divide into lobar bronchi, which subdivide into segmental bronchi.

Location of trachea and right and left mainstem bronchi

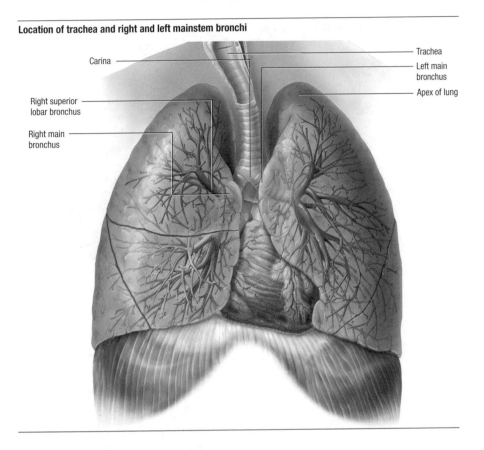

Location of larynx, epiglottis, and vocal cords

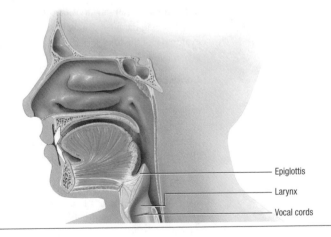

Location of terminal bronchioles and alveoli

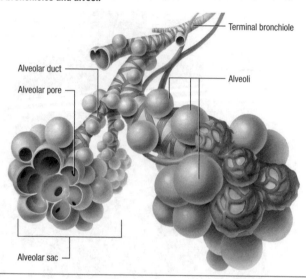

The airways continue to systematically branch, narrow, shorten, and increase in number toward the lung periphery. They divide about 25 times before ultimately opening into the terminal, or respiratory, bronchioles.

Terminal bronchioles

The terminal bronchioles, which have a few alveoli budding from their walls, branch into alveolar ducts that are completely lined with alveoli. Known as the *respiratory zone*, this area is where gas exchange occurs. These airways and their alveoli form the respiratory lobules of the lungs. The terminal bronchioles account for the last six or seven airway divisions. The distance from the terminal bronchiole to the most distal alveolus is only about 5 mm; however, most of the lung surface area available for gas exchange is contained in these spaces.

Conducting airways

The airways between the nose and the terminal bronchioles—called the *conducting airways*—lead inspired gas to the gas exchange regions of the lungs. About 150 cc of inspired air remains in the conducting airways during each breath. These airways, called *anatomic dead space*, aren't involved in gas exchange.

The large airways below the glottis contain cartilage, smooth muscle, elastic fibers, connective tissue, and mucous glands. Anteriorly, the trachea and mainstem bronchi are composed of 20 rings of U-shaped cartilage. The cartilage that opens posteriorly is connected by a band of smooth muscle and fibroelastic tissue. About 30% of the wall thickness in the mainstem and lobar bronchi is cartilage. This cartilage becomes irregular and platelike and eventually disappears in the smaller airways, which consist solely of smooth muscle and elastic fibers.

The mucous and bronchial glands located in the bronchial walls secrete a serous mucus blanket onto the inside airway walls. This secreted mucus forms a thin, sticky layer that lies atop ciliated columnar epithelial cells, which line nearly all of the respiratory tract between the larynx and the terminal bronchioles. The mucus layer traps foreign particles in the inspired air before they can enter the lungs. Cilia move in a wavelike motion, propelling the sticky mucus layer toward the pharynx where it can be coughed out or swallowed. Together, the mucus layer and cilia protect the lungs, acting as a major defense mechanism against inhaled particles.

Lung lobes

Each lung is divided into lobes. The right lung has three lobes: the upper, middle, and lower. The left lung has only an upper and a lower lobe. The lung's apex (superior aspect) is located near the clavicle, and its base (inferior aspect) is located near the diaphragm. (See *Lung lobes*, page 110.)

Alveoli

The terminal bronchioles divide into two to five alveolar ducts, each of which consists of 10 to 16 alveoli. Alveoli contain three cell types. Type I, the largest, is the lining cell and accounts for 95% of the alveolar surface area. The type II cell produces surfactant, a mixture of phospholipids. The macrophage, the third cell type, acts as a phagocytic defense mechanism against infection.

The adult respiratory system contains about 300 million alveoli. In a healthy adult, the surface area of the alveolar-capillary membrane available for O_2–CO_2 exchange is 70 to 85 m^2, about the size of a tennis court.

AGE ISSUE *Adults have about 10 times the number of alveoli as infants, who have alveoli that are larger with less elastic recoil. The number of alveoli reaches that of an adult by age 12.*

The alveolar surface is covered by a fluid layer containing surfactant. The surfactant mixes with pulmonary fluids and maintains alveolar stability by lowering the alveolar surface tension. This action protects against atelectasis and hypoxia by preventing the air-filled alveoli from collapsing at low volumes from the weight of capillary blood.

Lung lobes

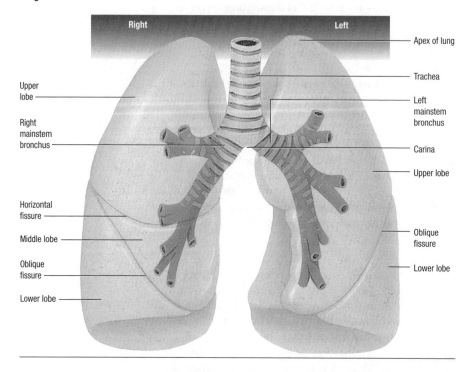

Lower airway innervation

Two neural pathways, the parasympathetic and sympathetic nervous systems, innervate the tracheobronchial tree. The relative balance of the two neural pathways and their effect on the smooth muscle, which lines the tracheobronchial tree, results in bronchial smooth muscle tone.

The parasympathetic nervous system in the larynx, trachea, and bronchi includes vagal nerve fibers and irritant receptors mediated by the neurotransmitter acetylcholine. Parasympathetic stimulation precipitates bronchoconstriction, coughing, and mucus discharge from the bronchial glands. Irritant receptors within the airways are believed to be responsible for increasing ventilation and precipitating coughing.

Sympathetic innervation of the lower airways usually arises from the thoracic nerves T1 through T5 and is mediated by the

Pulmonary circulation

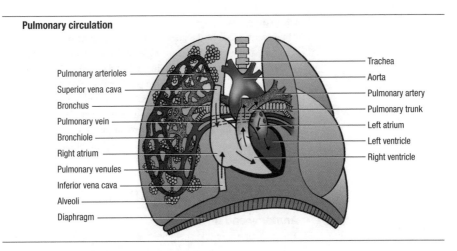

Pulmonary arterioles
Superior vena cava
Bronchus
Pulmonary vein
Bronchiole
Right atrium
Pulmonary venules
Inferior vena cava
Alveoli
Diaphragm

Trachea
Aorta
Pulmonary artery
Pulmonary trunk
Left atrium
Left ventricle
Right ventricle

postganglionic hormone transmitter norepinephrine. Sympathetic stimulation of beta$_2$-adrenergic receptors throughout the lower airways facilitates smooth muscle relaxation, resulting in bronchodilation.

The secretory mast cells on the surface of the large airways also may be stimulated or affected by drugs, hormones, antigens, and other messenger cells to precipitate or control bronchoconstriction.

Pulmonary and bronchial circulation

Two blood supplies, the pulmonary and bronchial circulations, facilitate gas exchange and nourish the airways and other lung tissues.

The pulmonary circulation begins as the pulmonary artery leaves the right ventricle. The pulmonary artery divides into segmental arteries, which subdivide, ending in the pulmonary capillary bed surrounding the alveoli. The capillaries then join to form venules, which converge to form veins, then pulmonary veins. The pulmonary veins end in the left atrium.

The bronchial circulation usually originates in the aorta and branches along the bronchi to provide oxygen and nutrients to the lung tissue and to clear metabolic wastes from the airways and other lung tissues. Oxygenated blood is pumped from the aorta to the tracheobronchial tree and travels through arterioles along the airways. Deoxygenated blood from the bronchial circulation is returned to the left atrium, accounting for the normal 2% to 3% right-to-left shunt.

Pleurae

The inner surface of the chest wall and the outer surface of the lungs are joined by thin, membranous tissues called the *pleurae*. The parietal pleura covers the inner surface of the chest wall, and the visceral pleura covers the outer surfaces of the lungs. A small amount of pleural fluid exists between the two layers. The pleurae separate into the right and left pleural cavities, which contain the lungs. During expansion and contraction of the chest wall and lungs, the pleurae glide smoothly and silently over each other.

THE MECHANICS OF BREATHING

Anatomy and physiology

The respiratory muscles help the chest cavity expand and contract. Pressure differences between atmospheric air and the lungs help produce air movement.

Thorax

The *thorax* is the bony structure that protects the vital organs (the heart and lungs) and permits chest expansion during inspiration. Twelve pairs of ribs are attached in a hingelike manner posteriorly to the vertebral column. This hingelike attachment allows the chest wall to be mobile during the respiratory cycle. The superior six pairs of ribs are attached anteriorly to the sternum.

Diaphragm

The *diaphragm*, the primary muscle of respiration, is composed of two dome-shaped hemidiaphragms that are attached to the lower edge of the rib cage. The right hemidiaphragm sits higher than the left. The diaphragm forms the inferior "floor" of the thorax. During inspiration, the diaphragm flattens and descends toward the abdomen. During expiration, it relaxes and ascends to its resting, dome-shaped configuration.

Intercostal muscles

Lying at right angles to each other, the internal and external intercostal muscles help to maintain the pressure difference between the pleurae and body surface. These muscles, located between the ribs and innervated by the intercostal nerves, contract during inspiration to stabilize, elevate, and expand the rib cage.

 AGE ISSUE *Children are diaphragmatic breathers until about age 6 because of their poorly developed intercostal muscles.*

Posterior view of thorax

Spinous process of C7

Scapula

First rib

Anterior view of thorax

First rib

Sternum

Accessory muscles of respiration

The *accessory muscles of respiration*—the sternocleidomastoid, scalene, trapezius, and rhomboid muscles—are involved in labored or forceful breathing. The sternocleidomastoid muscle elevates the sternum, increasing the anterior-to-posterior chest diameter. The scalene muscles elevate and fix the first two ribs. The trapezius and rhomboid muscles are activated during respiration but probably have no effect on forceful inspiration. The contraction of internal and external intercostal muscles may also be obvious in extremely labored breathing.

AGE ISSUE *Age-related anatomic changes that affect the respiratory system include increased anteroposterior diameter of the chest wall (reducing rib mobility and muscle contraction), increased chest wall stiffness with weakened diaphragmatic muscles (increasing use of accessory muscles), and elevated ribs and flattened diaphragm (decreasing chest expansion). Also, because of such factors as osteoporosis and vertebral collapse, kyphosis advances with age, decreasing lung expansion.*

Abdominal muscles

Abdominal muscles usually don't participate actively in relaxed breathing but play an important role during forceful expiratory efforts, such as coughing or sneezing. The internal intercostal muscles also contract forcefully during expiration.

Diaphragm during inspiration

Diaphragm

Diaphragm during expiration

Diaphragm

Normal breathing

During inspiration, the diaphragm and external intercostal muscles are activated. Diaphragmatic contraction flattens the domed diaphragm and expands the lower rib cage, forcing the abdominal contents downward and out, thus increasing the longitudinal lung size. The external intercostal muscle contraction stabilizes the rib cage and moves it outward and upward. The posterior cricoarytenoid muscle contracts to open the glottis. As the thorax expands, intrapleural pressures become subatmospheric, resulting in lung expansion and decreased intrapulmonary pressures. Inspired air flows from higher atmospheric pressure into the airways. At the end of inspiration, diaphragmatic movement declines and the air inflow gradually slows.

During expiration, the thorax and the elastic recoil force of the lungs return to their resting positions, increasing intrapleural pressures. This increased pressure forces air to flow out of the lower and upper airways. At the end of expiration, during quiet breathing, all muscles are relaxed and the diaphragm has returned to its resting position.

Distribution of ventilation and blood flow

During normal breathing in the upright position, air movement (ventilation) is greatest in the lung bases or dependent lung regions. Because of the pull of gravity, the alveoli in the lung bases collapse to a smaller size during expiration than do the alveoli in the lung apices. During inspiration, the alveoli in the lung bases open more easily, causing ventilation in the bases to be greater than in the apices.

 AGE ISSUE *In the older adult, airway closure and a loss of surface area results in decreased ventilation at the bases of the lungs.*

Gravity

Blood perfusion in the lungs also depends on gravity. The dependent lung regions receive a larger proportion of the cardiac output than the nondependent regions. When the patient is in the upright position, blood flow patterns in the apices are usually different from those in the bases. In the lung apices, alveolar (atmospheric) pressures exceed capillary hydrostatic pressure, and the capillaries remain partially collapsed during quiet breathing; this results in limited blood flow. In the lung bases, pulmonary arterial and venous hydrostatic pressures exceed atmospheric pressure, and the capillaries remain open throughout quiet breathing; this results in proportionately more blood flow to the lung bases than to the apices.

Posture

Postural changes affect the distribution of air and blood flow throughout the lungs. In the supine position, the apices and bases receive equal amounts of air and blood flow. In the lateral position, dependent lung regions receive more air and blood flow than nondependent regions.

Size and shape

The dimensions and shape of the tracheobronchial tree also affect the airflow pattern. During inspiration, air velocity and the airflow rate decrease as the total cross-sectional airway area increases with subsequent branching. Consequently, the larger airways conduct the same volume of air as do the more numerous smaller airways. This means that inspired air travels 100 times faster in the trachea than it does in the terminal bronchi.

Beyond the terminal bronchi, the forward movement of air is minimal. In the terminal bronchioles, diffusion is the primary method of air movement. The mean airflow velocity during

Anterior thoracic structures and landmark lines

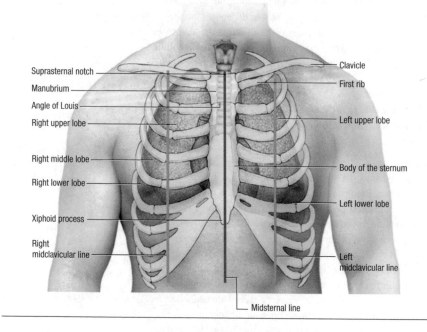

Suprasternal notch
Manubrium
Angle of Louis
Right upper lobe
Right middle lobe
Right lower lobe
Xiphoid process
Right midclavicular line
Clavicle
First rib
Left upper lobe
Body of the sternum
Left lower lobe
Left midclavicular line
Midsternal line

inspiration is about 100 m/second in the trachea but less than 1 cm/second in the terminal bronchioles.

AUSCULTATORY AREAS

Thoracic structures and landmarks
Accurate interpretation of breath sounds depends on a systematic approach to auscultation; it also requires the ability to describe the location of abnormal findings in relation to bony structures and anatomic landmark lines.

Breath sounds are auscultated over the anterior chest wall surface, the lateral chest wall surfaces, and the posterior chest wall surface.

Anterior chest wall surface
The lung apices extend ¼″ to 1½″ (2 to 4 cm) above the clavicles. The trachea bifurcates at the level of the sternal angle, the junction between the manubrium and the body of the sternum. The ribs and intercostal spaces provide precise horizontal landmarks to describe the location of breath sounds; the second rib and second intercostal space serve as reference points.

Posterior thoracic structures and landmark lines

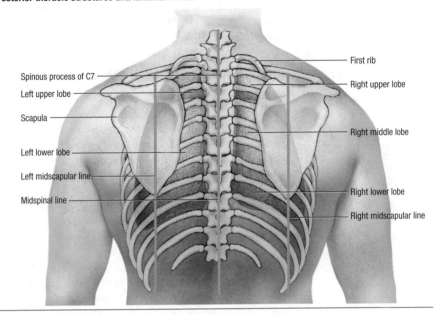

Spinous process of C7

Left upper lobe

Scapula

Left lower lobe

Left midscapular line

Midspinal line

First rib

Right upper lobe

Right middle lobe

Right lower lobe

Right midscapular line

Vertical landmark lines on the anterior chest wall surface include the midclavicular lines and the midsternal line. The right and left midclavicular lines extend downward from the center of each clavicle. The midsternal line bisects the sternum. The right lung base crosses the sixth rib at the right midclavicular line, and the left lung base crosses the seventh rib at the left midclavicular line.

Lateral chest wall surfaces

The lateral chest wall surfaces are also divided using landmark lines. The anterior axillary line extends downward from the anterior axillary fold, the midaxillary line extends downward from the apex of the axilla, and the posterior axillary line extends downward from the posterior axillary fold.

Posterior chest wall surface

Bony structures underlying the posterior chest wall surface also provide landmarks to locate breath sounds. The scapulae's inferior borders, located at about the same level as the seventh rib, serve as reference points. The numbered thoracic vertebrae provide horizontal landmarks.

 AUSCULTATION TIP *When auscultating the posterior chest wall, keep in mind that you'll be mostly hearing the lower lobes because of the anatomical positions of the lobes.*

Left lateral landmark lines

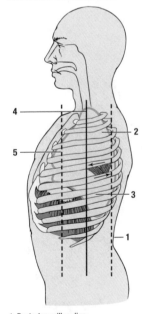

1. Posterior axillary line
2. Left upper lobe
3. Left lower lobe
4. Midaxillary line
5. Anterior axillary line

Landmark lines on the posterior chest wall surface provide vertical reference points. The midscapular lines extend downward from the inferior angle of each scapula, and the vertebral line extends downward over the vertebrae.

AUSCULTATORY TECHNIQUES

Using the stethoscope

The stethoscope allows you to hear breath sounds transmitted through the chest wall. Most stethoscopes have a diaphragm and a bell, with one or two tubes leading to the binaural headpiece and earpieces. The diaphragm is used to listen for high-pitched breath sounds; the bell is used to listen for low-pitched breath sounds. (See *Parts of the stethoscope*, page 9.) Applying the stethoscope firmly to the chest wall amplifies high-frequency sounds. However, if too much pressure is applied when using the bell, the stretched skin functions as a diaphragm and filters out low-pitched sounds.

The stethoscope tubing should be no longer than 10″ to 12″ (25 to 30 cm). It should be tightly attached to the binaural headpiece and the stethoscope body to prevent air leakage, which could result in the loss of sound energy. The earpieces must be securely attached to the binaural headpiece, which removes extraneous noise from the environment, to avoid any sound loss. They should fit tightly and should be placed into the ears in an anterior direction so that they conform to the direction of the ear canals.

AUSCULTATION TIP *Check the stethoscope to ensure that the diaphragm and bell are locked into place before auscultating. Some stethoscopes have a rotating bell or diaphragm that may become disengaged, which would block or muffle breath sounds.*

Listening to breath sounds

Breath sounds have a wide range of sound frequencies, many near the lower threshold of human hearing. Consequently, the environment for auscultation should be as quiet as possible so that you can hear breath sounds clearly and distinctly.

During auscultation, press the diaphragm of the stethoscope against the patient's chest wall over the intercostal spaces. Try not to listen directly over bone. Never listen through clothing, which impedes or alters sound transmission. Keep the stethoscope still and in place.

AUSCULTATION TIP *If the patient has a hairy chest or back, lightly dampen the chest and hold the stethoscope firmly against the skin to minimize the crackling noises produced by the hair.*

Auscultatory sequence

The auscultatory sequence for the posterior chest wall surface includes 10 different sites. (See *Posterior auscultatory sequence*, page 120.) The first site is above the left scapula over the lung apex. From there, the auscultatory sequence follows a pattern that progresses downward from the lung apices to the bases. This pattern covers the entire posterior chest wall surface and includes a comparison of sounds heard over the same auscultatory site over both the right and left lungs. Sites 5, 7, and 10 are located over the lateral chest wall surfaces.

The anterior chest wall auscultatory sequence includes nine sites and follows the same pattern as the posterior chest wall sequence. The pattern also includes sites over the lateral chest wall surfaces. (See *Anterior auscultatory sequence*, page 120.)

Comparing breath sounds

If the patient is alert and healthy, begin auscultation with the patient sitting upright and leaning slightly forward. Position yourself behind the patient. Ask the patient to breathe through an open mouth, slightly deeper than usual, through several respiratory cycles. (*Note:* If the patient is extremely dyspneic, don't ask him to take deeper breaths. In this case, begin auscultating for breath sounds at the bilateral lung bases.) Place the diaphragm of the stethoscope over the left lung apex, and listen for at least one complete respiratory cycle. Then move the diaphragm to the same site over the right lung. Compare the breath sounds heard over these same locations. Continue in this manner, making contralateral comparisons at each auscultatory site.

After auscultating the entire posterior chest wall and parts of the lateral chest walls, move to the front of the patient. Have the patient place his arms at his sides and breathe through an open mouth, slightly deeper than usual, as you listen to breath sounds over the anterior chest wall. You can obtain additional information about tracheal sounds by auscultating over the sternum, larynx, and mouth.

 AUSCULTATION TIP *You may roll patients who are comatose, critically ill, or bedridden from one side to another to auscultate dependent lung regions. Listen initially over dependent lung regions because gravity-dependent secretions or fluids may produce abnormal sounds that sometimes disappear when the patient is turned, breathes deeply, or coughs.*

Posterior auscultatory sequence

Anterior auscultatory sequence

AUSCULTATION TIP *To gain the trust and cooperation of a child, allow him to listen to your lungs or to a stuffed animal or doll.*

◀◀◀POSTTEST

1. What is the primary function of the respiratory system?
2. Describe the anatomy of the lower airway from the mainstem bronchi to the alveoli.
3. Where are the apex and base of the lung located?
4. Describe normal breathing.
5. How are air and blood distributed in the lungs?
6. Name the anatomic structures and landmark lines on the anterior chest wall surface.
7. Name the anatomic structures and landmark lines on the lateral chest wall surface.
8. Name the anatomic structures and landmark lines on the posterior chest wall surface.
9. How is the stethoscope used to auscultate for breath sounds?
10. Describe the sequence used during auscultation to compare breath sounds.

Introduction to Breath Sounds

BREATH SOUND PRODUCTION

Three types of sounds are heard during auscultation—normal breath sounds, abnormal breath sounds (including voice sounds), and adventitious sounds. Breath sounds are produced by airflow patterns, by associated pressure changes within the airways, and by solid tissue vibrations within the lungs. Both normal and abnormal breath sounds have certain recognizable characteristics. Their intensity, duration, frequency, and quality are believed to be affected by airflow patterns, regional lung volume or distribution of air, body position, and the sound production site.

The sounds are normally diminished and filtered when they are transmitted through air-filled alveoli, fluid accumulations in the pleura, and solid structures, such as bone.

Breath sound origination

The sites where normal breath sounds originate aren't clearly defined. For example, sounds heard over the trachea and large airways are characterized as high-pitched, harsh, loud, and tubular (hollow) with a long expiratory phase. These sounds are thought to reflect the turbulent airflow patterns in the first divisions of the large airways.

Sounds heard over other chest wall areas are softer and have a shorter expiratory phase. These sounds may also be produced by turbulent airflow in the first few divisions of the large airways; however, the fact that these sounds vary with changing airflow rates and distribution of ventilation in the lungs suggests that they are produced in the peripheral airways. Also, inspiratory sounds may be produced in the peripheral airways, and expiratory sounds may be produced in the larger airways. Breath sounds aren't produced in the terminal bronchioles because of minimal airflow rates.

Disease

Disease processes that alter the airway or airflow dynamics produce abnormal breath sounds or adventitious sounds. These sounds are generated by the vibration of solid structures, by airflow through narrowed airways, or by abrupt changes in airway pressure.

Airway dynamics

The stability of an airway depends on the interaction of the elastic properties of the lung tissue, the intrapulmonary airways, and the pressures—both internal and external—exerted on the airways. During the respiratory cycle, a pressure gradient exists across the airway wall and between the trachea and alveoli. As the chest expands during inspiration, intrapleural pressure falls. At the same time, the lung's elastic recoil increases, exerting traction on airway walls. This traction increases the airway's diameter and decreases the resistance to airflow. The pressure gradient between the alveolar and atmospheric pressures increases, driving air through the airways toward the alveoli.

AGE ISSUE *In older persons, pulmonary function decreases because of respiratory muscle degeneration or atrophy. Ventilatory capacity diminishes because the lungs' diffusing capacity declines, decreased inspiratory and expiratory muscle strength diminishes vital capacity, and lung tissue degeneration causes a decrease in the lungs' elastic recoil capacity, which results in an elevated residual volume. For these reasons, aging can cause changes consistent with emphysema.*

Intrapleural pressure and alveolar elastic recoil pressures drive expiratory airflow. At the beginning of expiration, intrapleural pressure and the alveolar recoil force cause the alveolar pressures to rise and push the air through the airways and out through the upper airway. Air pressures fall as the air flows through the airways from the alveoli to the upper airway. A point is reached, particularly during forceful expiration, when intrapleural and intrapulmonary pressures are equal. Called the *equal pressure point*, it can occur anywhere within the thorax and is a function of the mechanical properties of the lung (elastic recoil, airflow resistance, and stiffness of the walls of the airway). Downstream from this point, pressures outside of the airways can compress and further narrow the airways, causing increased resistance to airflow.

Airflow patterns

Variations in airflow patterns are affected by the intricate network of branching airways, the various airway diameters, and the potential for irregular airway wall surfaces within the tracheobronchial tree.

Turbulent airflow	Transitional airflow	Laminar airflow

Turbulent airflow

During rapid, or *turbulent*, airflow, air molecules move randomly, colliding against airway walls and each other. They may move across or against the general direction of airflow. The colliding air molecules produce rapid pressure changes within the airway, and these rapid pressure changes produce sounds. Turbulent airflow occurs in the trachea, mainstem bronchi, and other larger airways.

Transitional airflow

As airflow is forced to change directions abruptly in the branching airways, the airstream separates into layers and moves at different velocities.

Laminar airflow

In the terminal or small airways and respiratory bronchioles, airflow is slow and laminar, or *nonturbulent*. No abrupt changes in pressure or airway wall movements occur to generate sound. Consequently, air movement in these areas produces no sound.

Mechanical vibrations

Breath sounds are also produced by mechanical vibrations of solid tissue. These vibrations travel through the different media of air, fluid, or tissue at varying speeds. Their frequency, intensity, and duration can be measured.

Frequency

Frequency, measured in hertz (Hz), refers to the number of vibrations occurring per unit of time. Different frequencies produce the different sounds heard during auscultation. In the clinical setting, the term *pitch* is used to describe sound frequency. High-pitched sounds have higher frequencies; low-pitched sounds, lower frequencies.

Intensity

Intensity, the loudness or softness of the vibrations producing breath sounds, can be measured electronically by recording amplitude. Intensity is affected by the type of vibrating structure producing the sound, the distance the sound travels, and the transmission pathway.

Duration

The duration of the vibrations that produce breath sounds can be measured in milliseconds. However, the human ear perceives sounds during auscultation as long or short and as continuous or discontinuous.

Sound damping

Body structures or cavities that produce resonance selectively transmit or amplify breath sounds that are similar in frequency and absorb, or damp, those with other frequencies. Breath sounds arising from the same location in the lung have a higher pitch when heard at the mouth or over the trachea than when heard over the chest wall. This change in pitch occurs because high-pitched breath sounds are absorbed as they're transmitted through the lungs and thorax.

Voice sounds are also affected by damping. The resonant qualities of the mouth, nasopharynx, paranasal sinuses, and chest cavity contribute to the pitch and intensity of voice sounds.

Impedance matching

Breath and voice sounds are normally damped when they're transmitted through air, fluid, and tissue. However, when these sounds are transmitted sequentially through media with different acoustic properties, the sounds' vibrations are filtered and reflected at the interface of the different media. The amount of filtering that takes place depends on the media's impedance (resistance to sound transmission).

Impedance match

When two media are matched according to acoustic properties, sound is transmitted effectively. For example, consolidated areas enhance the transmission of breath sounds to the chest wall. This happens because the consolidating substance, an inflammatory exudate, collects in alveoli, replacing air with dense lung tissue. Consequently, the fluid-filled, airless lung tissue and the chest wall are acoustically well-matched, and breath sounds are transmitted more easily.

Impedance mismatch

The transmission of breath and voice sounds through either tissue or fluid between inflated lung segments and the chest wall results in an impedance mismatch. The vibrations of the sounds are significantly filtered and reflected back to their source by the pleurae. Diseases that increase the impedance mismatch, such as a large pleural effusion or empyema, diminish breath sound intensity. Obesity also is associated with diminished breath sounds because of the increased distance between the stethoscope and the lungs.

 AUSCULTATION TIP *For better results when auscultating the lungs of a patient who's obese, ask him to take deep breaths through his open mouth while sitting upright or standing.*

TERMINOLOGY

Classifying breath sounds
Normal breath sounds are classified as tracheal, bronchial, vesicular, or bronchovesicular. Tracheal and bronchial sounds, produced by turbulent airflow, are loud and can be heard throughout inspiration and expiration over the trachea and mainstem bronchi. (◆Sound 51) Vesicular breath sounds are faint; they're best heard over other chest wall areas throughout inspiration and at the beginning of expiration. (◆Sound 52)

Bronchovesicular breath sounds are heard over areas between the mainstem bronchi and the smaller airways; their pitch and duration are midway between those of tracheal and mainstem bronchi breath sounds and normal breath sounds heard over other chest wall areas. (◆Sound 53) Bronchovesicular sounds are heard during inspiration and expiration for equal amounts of time.

Classifying voice sounds
Voice sounds are vibrations produced by speech that are transmitted to the chest wall through the tracheobronchial tree. Voice sounds are classified as bronchophony, egophony, and whispered pectoriloquy.

Voice sounds auscultated over the chest wall are called *bronchophony*. In a healthy individual, bronchophony is similar to voice sounds heard through the neck. (◆Sound 54) Voice sounds transmitted through the chest wall that have selectively amplified higher-pitched frequencies are called *egophony*. (◆Sound 55) High-pitched whispered sounds transmitted through airless, consolidated lung tissue are called *whispered pectoriloquy*. (◆Sound 56)

Classifying adventitious sounds
Adventitious sounds are added sounds that are heard with normal and abnormal breath sounds. They're classified as either crackles or wheezes and then further classified by duration and pitch. (See Chapter 18 for a further discussion of adventitious breath sound terminology.)

DOCUMENTING AUSCULTATION FINDINGS

Careful documentation of auscultation findings is necessary to determine if the sounds heard have changed over time. This requires the same systematic approach used during auscultation. First, determine the location, intensity, duration, and pitch of each sound during auscultation, and then document these characteristics in the patient's record.

Location

Document sound location by describing anatomic thoracic landmarks and indicating the anterior, posterior, or lateral chest wall surface where the sound is heard.

 AGE ISSUE *Because the chest wall of the neonate is very thin, sound is transmitted throughout all lung fields, making it difficult to pinpoint its origin.*

You can also document *location* by using the lung bases or apices as reference points. Also document whether the sounds are heard bilaterally (over both lungs) or unilaterally (over one lung).

Intensity

Sound *intensity* is described subjectively, using such terms as *loud, soft, absent, diminished*, or *distant*.

Duration

Sound *duration* refers to the sound's timing within the respiratory cycle—that is, whether it's heard during inspiration, expiration, or both. Timing can be described as early, late, or prolonged.

Pitch

Sound *pitch* is usually described as high or low. Documenting pitch is more important when wheezes or crackles have been noted during auscultation because pitch helps differentiate the underlying disease process.

Putting them all together

A typical documentation example might read: "Late inspiratory fine crackles were heard over the right base posteriorly along the midscapular line, and coarse crackles were heard throughout inspiration and expiration over the left apex anteriorly near the midclavicular line." Such a description provides the reader with valuable information about any adventitious sounds heard during auscultation.

◀◀◀ POSTTEST

1. How are breath sounds produced?
2. Briefly describe the differences between breath sounds heard over the trachea and mainstem bronchi and those heard over other chest wall areas.
3. Describe turbulent airflow.
4. Describe vortices.
5. Describe laminar airflow.
6. What is meant by frequency, intensity, and duration of breath sounds?
7. Compare and contrast tracheal and mainstem bronchi breath sounds with normal breath sounds heard over other chest wall areas.
8. Define the terms *bronchophony*, *egophony*, and *whispered pectoriloquy*.
9. What are adventitious sounds?
10. Name the four characteristics used to describe breath sounds.

Normal breath sounds

14 Breath sounds heard in healthy individuals

PRETEST ◆◆◆

1. What are normal breath sounds?
2. How do normal breath sounds originate?
3. What affects the normal breath sound characteristics?
4. What is the significance of breath sounds heard at the mouth?

ANATOMY AND PHYSIOLOGY

Normal breath sounds are broadly defined as breathing heard through the chest wall of a healthy person. They include tracheal, bronchial, vesicular, and bronchovesicular sounds, as well as sounds heard at the mouth. Three variables affect the normal sounds heard during auscultation: the distance between the source of the sound and the chest wall, the path of sound transmission, and the sound's location. Normal breath sounds are produced by airflow patterns, by associated pressure changes within the airways, and by solid tissue vibrations.

Normal breath sounds heard over large airways are produced by turbulent airflow in those airways. They're loudest when auscultated over the trachea on the anterior chest wall surface next to the sternum. As air travels through the airways beyond the segmental bronchi, these normally high-pitched sounds become diminished because they're filtered by the chest wall, pleurae, and air-filled lung tissue. The normal breath sounds heard over most of the chest wall surface are soft and low-pitched; they're softer and shorter during expiration than during inspiration.

Tracheal and bronchial breath sounds

Normal breath sounds heard over the trachea (tracheal breath sounds) (◆**Sound 51**) and mainstem bronchi (bronchial breath sounds) are produced by turbulent airflow patterns. Tracheal breath sounds are described as harsh and high-pitched and can be heard over the trachea. Bronchial breath sounds (◆**Sound 57**) are described as loud and high-pitched and can be heard next to the trachea. Inspired and expired air travels easily through these large airways.

Airway area producing tracheal and mainstem bronchi breath sounds

1. Trachea
2. Right mainstem bronchus
3. Left mainstem bronchus

Auscultatory sites for normal breath sounds heard over other chest wall areas

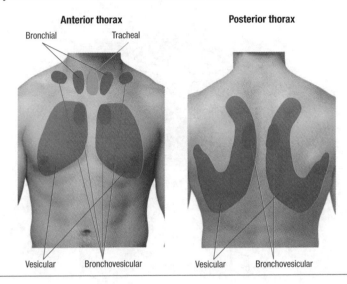

| Anterior thorax | Posterior thorax |

Bronchial Tracheal

Vesicular Bronchovesicular Vesicular Bronchovesicular

When tracheal breath sounds are being auscultated, a brief pause may be heard at the end of inspiration, and expiration is longer than inspiration. (◆**Sound 57**) The inspiratory–expiratory (I:E) ratio is 1:2 to 1:3. The sound frequency distribution of these breath sounds is 200 to 2,000 Hz. (◆**Sound 57**)

Tracheal and mainstem bronchi (bronchial) breath sounds are heard over the chest wall on either side of the sternum from the second intercostal space to the fourth intercostal space anteriorly and along the vertebral column from the third intercostal space to the sixth intercostal space posteriorly. These sounds have a variable pitch and a loud intensity heard best using the diaphragm of the stethoscope; they're heard throughout inspiration and expiration. (See *Auscultatory sites for tracheal and mainstem bronchi breath sounds*, page 132.)

Vesicular breath sounds

Vesicular breath sounds are transmitted through lung tissue and the chest wall and are produced by changes in airflow patterns. These normal sounds are quieter than tracheal and bronchial sounds. Inspiration is heard clearly, and expiration immediately follows inspiration but quickly fades as airflow rates rapidly decline and turbulent airflow is directed toward the central airways. The I:E ratio is 3:1 to 4:1. The sound frequency distribution of these normal breath sounds is 200 to 600 Hz. (◆**Sounds 58 and 59**)

Airway areas producing vesicular breath sounds

Auscultatory sites for tracheal and mainstem bronchi breath sounds

Anterior view

Posterior view

Bronchovesicular breath sounds

Bronchovesicular breath sounds are heard anteriorly and posteriorly over the central large airways. Their pitch and duration are midway between those of the vesicular breath sounds and the bronchial sounds; inspiratory and expiratory phases are equal, with an I:E ratio of 1:1.

 ***AGE ISSUE** Bronchovesicular breath sounds may be heard in the outer fields in children as old as age 6 because infants and young children have thin chest walls and muscles that don't diminish breath sounds to the same extent as the thicker chest walls of adults.*

Variations in intensity

The intensity of bronchovesicular breath sounds changes during deep inspiration and after maximal expiration. The intensity may also change depending on the lung area being auscultated. For example, if the patient is sitting up during auscultation of the anterior chest wall surface, breath sounds are louder over the apices during early inspiration and become progressively softer as inspiration continues. (♦**Sound 59**) During auscultation of the posterior lung bases, breath sounds are initially softer and become progressively louder during maximal inspiration.

Variations in intensity are usually related to airflow patterns and to the distribution of air throughout the lungs. During inspiration with the patient in the upright position, air flows initially into the lung apices, then into the lung bases (the dependent areas) after the small airways reopen; therefore, the intensity will probably be greater in the apices than in the bases. During normal breathing, this change in intensity may not always be audible.

Variations in intensity that are unrelated to airflow rates or regional ventilation may be heard when comparing symmetrical sites on the chest wall. For example, breath sounds heard over the left lower lobe may vary in intensity with the cardiac cycle. The intensity may increase during systole because ventricular contraction allows the surrounding lung tissue to expand more fully, increasing turbulent airflow to that region and intensifying the inspiratory sounds. Conversely, the intensity may decrease during diastole because ventricular expansion of the heart compresses adjacent lung tissue, reducing airflow to that region.

Bronchovesicular breath sounds have a low pitch that can be heard using either the diaphragm or bell of the stethoscope. They're softer and less harsh than bronchial breath sounds and have a tubular quality. (♦**Sound 58**)

Normal breath sounds heard at the mouth

Normal breath sounds heard at the mouth are thought to be produced by turbulent airflow occurring below the glottis and before the terminal airways. In healthy individuals, breath sounds at the

Airway area producing normal breath sounds heard at mouth

mouth provide baseline data that can be useful later when evaluating noisy or paradoxically quiet breath sounds.

Normal breath sounds heard at the mouth are heard at the lips. Their intensity is as loud and harsh as that of tracheal and mainstem bronchi breath sounds, and their duration is continuous (throughout the respiratory cycle). They have a moderately high pitch.

◀◀◀ POSTTEST

1. Define normal breath sounds.
2. What variables affect the normal breath sounds heard during auscultation?
3. How are normal breath sounds produced?
4. Describe tracheal and mainstem bronchi breath sounds.
5. Describe the breath sounds heard over other chest wall areas.
6. How do ventilation and airflow rate changes affect breath sound intensity?
7. How do cardiac systole and diastole affect normal breath sound intensity?
8. How are breath sounds heard at the mouth produced?

Abnormal breath sounds

CHAPTER 15

Bronchial breath sounds

PRETEST ▶▶▶

1. What happens to normal breath sounds when lung density increases?
2. What are bronchial breath sounds?
3. How does consolidation affect breath sounds?
4. How does atelectasis affect breath sounds?
5. How does fibrosis affect breath sounds?

SOUND PRODUCTION

When lung tissue between the central airways and the chest wall becomes airless because of conditions that increase lung density, transmission of breath sounds from large airways is enhanced. This happens because little high-frequency sound is lost through attenuation or filtration. As lung tissue density increases the impedance between the fluid-filled lung tissue and the pleurae and chest wall, these three media become well-matched, which decreases the normal filtering of high-frequency sounds. Consequently, breath sounds are transmitted more readily to the chest wall surface and are louder and more tubular than normal breath sounds heard over the same chest wall area. Expiration is significantly louder and longer than normal. The inspiratory–expiratory (I:E) ratio changes from the normal 3:1 or 4:1 to 1:1 or 1:2. These sounds, called *bronchial breath sounds*, are considered abnormal when found anywhere except anteriorly over the large airways.

Related conditions

Conditions associated with bronchial breath sounds include consolidation, atelectasis, and fibrosis, all of which increase lung tissue density because of fluid accumulation, lung collapse, or fibrotic scarring. Bronchial breath sounds are heard over the affected lung area.

Consolidation

The most common cause of lung tissue consolidation (solidification) is pneumonia, a lung inflammation that can be caused by bacteria, viruses, or chemical insults (such as with aspiration). In this condition, fluid, leukocytes, and erythrocytes accumulate in spaces that are normally air-filled, producing a consolidated area. Clinical findings vary, depending on the location of the consolidated area and the causative agent. When classic consolidation is present, decreased chest wall movement and a dull percussion note are apparent over the affected area. Bronchial breath sounds are heard over a dense, airless *upper* lobe, even without a patent bronchus (◆**Sound 60**), because the upper lobe surfaces are in direct contact with the trachea and loud tracheal breath sounds are transmitted directly to the dense, airless upper lobe tissues. In contrast, bronchial breath sounds are heard over a dense, airless lower lobe only when the bronchi are patent, because sound isn't transmitted directly to the airless lower lobe tissues.

Sound characteristics
In a patient with lobar pneumonia with right posterior midlung consolidation, bronchial breath sounds are heard over the right posterior midlung field, located over the seventh and eighth intercostal spaces along the vertebral column. (See *Bronchial breath sounds heard over consolidated right posterior midlung*, page 138.) These sounds are high-pitched and have the typical hollow, or tubular, quality of normal central airway breath sounds. They remain audible during both expiration and inspiration, but the expiratory sounds are longer and louder when the patient is sitting up; the I:E ratio is 1:2. These sounds may be auscultated using either the bell or diaphragm of the stethoscope. (◆**Sound 60**)

Atelectasis
Atelectasis, incomplete expansion of a lung area, is typically diagnosed in postoperative or immobile patients and in some patients with bronchiectasis or pneumonia. It's thought to result from prolonged shallow breathing (hypoventilation) or uncleared secretions that occlude the airway. Because no air enters the distal airways, the segmental or lobar bronchi collapse. If a large airway is occluded, clinical findings include decreased chest wall movement, a dull percussion note, regional changes in lung volume, and bronchial breath sounds over a dense, airless upper airway. (◆**Sound 61**) However, decreased chest wall movement and lung volume changes may be difficult to detect on clinical examination.

Sound characteristics
Bronchial breath sounds are heard over an atelectatic area when the bronchus is patent. They aren't heard over an atelectatic lower lobe if the bronchus is obstructed.

In an unresponsive patient with a head injury, bronchial breath sounds are heard over the right anterior midlung field, located between the third and fifth intercostal spaces from the midsternal line to just right of the midclavicular line. These sounds are high-pitched and have the typical hollow, or tubular, quality of normal central airway breath sounds. They're audible throughout inspiration and expiration. When the patient is in the supine position, the inspiratory and expiratory sounds are equal in duration and intensity; the I:E ratio is 1:1. These sounds can be

Bronchial breath sounds heard over consolidated right posterior midlung

Affected lung area

Posterior auscultatory sites

heard equally well using either the bell or diaphragm of the stethoscope. (◆**Sound 61**)

Fibrosis

Severe fibrosis (abnormal formation of fibrous connective tissue) may produce bronchial breath sounds that are usually heard over the lower lung regions. Some possible causes of pulmonary fibrosis include smoke inhalation and exposure to asbestos. In most cases, however, the cause is unknown. The breath sounds heard over fibrotic areas are similar to those heard over atelectatic areas. (◆**Sound 62**)

Bronchial breath sounds heard over atelectatic right anterior midlung

Affected lung area

Anterior auscultatory sites

Sound characteristics

In some patients with asbestosis, bronchial breath sounds are heard anteriorly and posteriorly over both lung bases.

Anteriorly, this area extends from the midsternal line to the right and left of the anterior axillary lines over the fifth and sixth intercostal spaces; posteriorly, it extends from the vertebral line to the right and left of the posterior axillary lines over the seventh, eighth, ninth, and tenth intercostal spaces. (See *Auscultatory sites for asbestosis in lung bases*, page 140.)

Lung area affected by asbestosis

Auscultatory sites for asbestosis in lung bases

Anterior view

Posterior view

Because the bronchi are patent, bronchial breath sounds heard over fibrotic areas have the typical hollow, or tubular, quality of normal central airway breath sounds. They're audible throughout inspiration and expiration. When the patient is in the upright position, the breath sounds become progressively louder during inspiration and become both louder and longer during expiration; the I:E ratio is 1:1 to 1:2. These bronchial breath sounds are high-pitched and are heard equally well with either the diaphragm or bell of the stethoscope. **(◆Sound 62)**

◀◀◀POSTTEST

1. What happens when lung tissue becomes airless because of conditions that increase lung density?
2. Why are breath sounds enhanced over an area of increased lung density?
3. Name three conditions associated with bronchial breath sounds.
4. Which clinical findings are typically associated with consolidation?
5. What role does a patent bronchus have in the transmission of breath sounds to the apex and base of the lung?
6. Describe the characteristics of bronchial breath sounds heard over a consolidated area.
7. What causes atelectasis?
8. Describe the characteristics of bronchial breath sounds heard over an atelectatic area.
9. Describe the characteristics of bronchial breath sounds heard over a fibrotic area.

PRETEST ▶▶▶

1. How are normal voice sounds produced?
2. Name the three voice sounds.
3. How do voice sounds change over areas of dense, airless lung tissue?
4. Which specific words or letters is the patient asked to repeat to detect changes in bronchophony and egophony?
5. Which auscultatory findings are associated with consolidation?

SOUND PRODUCTION

Voice sounds are produced by vibrations of the vocal cords as air from the lungs passes over them. The resonance of the mouth, nasopharynx, and paranasal sinuses helps to amplify these sounds. When voice sounds pass through normally inflated, air-filled lungs, vowel tones, which contain many high-frequency sounds, are diminished and filtered. Like other high-frequency sounds, voice sounds are also selectively reflected back toward the lung tissue at the pleurae. Consequently, transmitted voice sounds are normally heard as a low-pitched, unintelligible mumble over healthy lung and pleural surfaces because most of the vowels are filtered out; conversely, they're heard distinctly over consolidated or atelectatic lung tissue areas because less filtering takes place, enhancing transmission.

Three types

The three types of voice sounds are bronchophony, whispered pectoriloquy, and egophony.

Bronchophony

Bronchophony is the clear, distinct, intelligible voice sound heard over dense, airless lung tissue. (◆Sound 63) Dense, airless lung tissue transmits high-frequency vowel sounds more easily because of impedance matching. Also, consolidation increases vocal resonance, which allows the clear transmission of voice sounds to the chest wall. Bronchophony is heard over dense, airless upper lobes because the upper lobe surfaces are in direct contact with the

Auscultatory sites for bronchophony heard over consolidated left upper lobe

Anterior view

Posterior view

trachea, leading to direct transmission of tracheal breath sounds. In contrast, bronchophony is heard over dense, airless lower lobes only when the bronchi are patent because a direct path of sound transmission to the lower lobes doesn't exist.

Sound characteristics

Bronchophony can be heard anywhere over the anterior, lateral, and posterior chest wall surfaces. It's commonly heard over dense, airless lung tissue in the upper lobes, such as a consolidated area. In a patient with left upper lobe pneumonia, intelligible voice sounds are heard over both the anterior and the posterior chest wall surfaces. The anterior area is located between the space above the clavicle and the second intercostal space from the

Consolidated lung area producing bronchophony in left upper lobe

Auscultatory sites for whispered pectoriloquy heard over atelectatic left lower lobe

Anterior view

Posterior view

Atelectatic lung area producing whispered pectoriloquy in lower left lobe

midsternal line to the left of the midclavicular line. The posterior area is located between the first and third intercostal spaces from the vertebral line toward the left midscapular line.

The patient is asked to repeat the words "ninety-nine" several times. Over healthy lung tissue, the words are unintelligible **(♦Sound 64)**; over a consolidated area, however, the high-frequency sounds are easily understood as words. **(♦Sound 65)**

Whispered pectoriloquy

Whispered pectoriloquy is the clear, distinct, intelligible whispered voice sound heard over airless, consolidated, or atelectatic lung tissue. In a healthy person, normal lung tissue filters the high frequencies of whispered vowel sounds, making them unintelligible during auscultation. In a patient with consolidation or atelectasis, these same whispered vowel sounds are transmitted to the chest wall surface without much filtering of high frequencies and can be heard clearly with the stethoscope. (♦**Sound 66**)

Sound characteristics

Whispered pectoriloquy can be heard anywhere over the anterior or posterior chest wall surfaces over dense, airless lung tissue, typically over an area of consolidation or atelectasis. In a post-operative patient with left lower lobe atelectasis and a patent bronchus, intelligible voice sounds are heard over the anterior and posterior chest wall surfaces. The anterior area is located over the fifth and sixth intercostal spaces from the midsternal line to the midaxillary line. The posterior area is located over the eighth, ninth, and tenth intercostal spaces from the vertebral line to the midaxillary line.

The patient is asked to whisper words such as "one-two-three" several times. Over healthy lung tissue, the words are unintelligible (♦**Sound 67**); over the atelectatic area, the high-frequency vowel sounds are easily understood as words. (♦**Sound 66**)

Egophony

Egophony, a voice sound that has a nasal or bleating quality when heard over the chest wall (♦**Sound 68**), is produced over consolidated and atelectatic areas because impedance matching enhances breath sound transmission in such areas. It's also detectable over the upper border of large pleural effusions.

Sound characteristics

Egophony can be heard anywhere over the anterior, posterior, or lateral chest wall surfaces over a consolidated or atelectatic area. In a patient with right lower lobe pneumonia, egophony is heard over the lateral chest wall surface. This area is located over the fifth and sixth intercostal spaces between the anterior axillary line and the midaxillary line.

The patient is asked to say the letter "E" several times. Over healthy lung tissue, the letter sounds as it normally does (♦**Sound 69**); over the consolidated area, it sounds like "A-aay" and has a high-pitched, nasal quality. (♦**Sound 68**)

Constellation of findings

A constellation of auscultatory findings—bronchial breath sounds, bronchophony, whispered pectoriloquy, and egophony—is typical in patients with consolidation. Bronchophony may be easier to hear when bronchial breath sounds are pronounced and consolidation is present in only one lobe or lung. Whispered pectoriloquy is typically discernible over atelectatic lung segments or areas of patchy consolidation where bronchial sounds or bronchophony isn't completely audible.

Consolidated lung area producing egophony in right lower lobe

◀◀◀ POSTTEST

1. How are voice sounds produced?
2. Describe the voice sounds heard over normal lung and pleural surfaces.
3. What happens to the voice sounds heard over a consolidated area or an atelectatic area?
4. Describe the characteristics of bronchophony.
5. Which words is the patient asked to repeat to detect changes in bronchophony?
6. Describe the characteristics of whispered pectoriloquy.
7. How is egophony produced over dense, airless lung tissue?
8. Describe the characteristics of egophony.
9. Which letter is the patient asked to repeat to detect changes in egophony?
10. What constellation of auscultatory findings is typical in patients with consolidation?

Absent and diminished breath sounds

CHAPTER 17

PRETEST ▶▶▶

1. Which conditions are associated with diminished or absent breath sounds?
2. How does each of these conditions cause diminished or absent breath sounds?
3. Does lung hyperinflation cause diminished or absent breath sounds?
4. How does positive end-expiratory pressure (PEEP) change the normal breath sound characteristics?
5. Does obesity change the normal breath sound characteristics?

SOUND PRODUCTION

Breath sounds are diminished or eliminated by conditions that limit airflow into lung segments. Slow inspiratory airflow rates decrease breath sound amplitude because less air movement occurs, resulting in less turbulent airflow.

Diminished or absent breath sounds can also occur when breath sounds are reflected at the visceral and parietal pleurae because of an impedance mismatch. A mismatch occurs when sounds are transmitted through two types of media with significantly different acoustical properties. For example, when breath sounds, which are normally transmitted through aerated lung tissue, are transmitted through a collection of fluid or air in the pleural space, sound transmission is halted or filtered. The same acoustical mismatch also occurs in patients with increased chest wall thickness. For example, in obese patients, breath sounds are diminished because they're transmitted through a layer of adipose tissue.

Normal turbulent airflow

Related conditions

Conditions associated with absent or diminished breath sounds include shallow breathing, diaphragmatic paralysis, airway obstruction, pneumothorax, pleural effusion, hyperinflated lungs, and obesity. The use of PEEP during assisted ventilation also is associated with diminished breath sounds.

Decreased **turbulent airflow in shallow breathing**

Shallow breathing

During normal breathing in the upright position, a certain amount of air flows through the airways during inspiration and expiration; the distribution of ventilation is greater in dependent lung regions because more respiratory movement occurs. During shallow breathing, less respiratory movement occurs; consequently, less air flows through the airways during inspiration and expiration. Because of this reduced airflow, turbulence is decreased and breath sounds are diminished. **(♦Sound 70)**

Sound characteristics

Diminished breath sounds may be heard over the anterior, posterior, and lateral chest wall surfaces. Postoperative patients and patients with rib fractures commonly breathe shallowly because pain limits their depth of respiration. Patients with decreased levels of consciousness from central nervous system injuries or drug overdoses may also have shallow breathing.

Diaphragmatic paralysis

During inspiration in a healthy person, contraction of the dome-shaped diaphragm expands the lower rib cage, forcing the abdominal contents downward and out and increasing the longitudinal lung size. Thoracic expansion lowers the intrapulmonary pressure, which allows air to flow into the airways.

When the diaphragm becomes paralyzed, as might happen with injury to the phrenic nerves, it no longer participates in normal breathing. The internal and external intercostal muscles, which also have a role in normal breathing, must take over the work of breathing. With only the chest wall muscles initiating the respiratory cycle, ventilation of the lung bases may be limited, resulting in diminished breath sounds.

Sound characteristics

Diminished sounds may be heard over the anterior, posterior, and lateral chest wall surfaces. **(♦Sound 71)**

 ALERT *In a patient with diaphragmatic paralysis, who has greatly diminished breath sounds, assess for respiratory distress and prepare for intubation and mechanical ventilation.*

Airway obstruction

An obstruction in an airway blocks the flow of air and, therefore, changes the breath sounds heard during auscultation. The location of the obstruction determines where the changes in breath sounds are heard.

Sound characteristics

If a lobar or segmental bronchus becomes obstructed, as in a patient who has aspirated a foreign object or one who has a large mucus plug, airflow ceases distal to the obstruction; therefore, breath sounds are absent over the area distal to the obstruction.

Lobar bronchus obstruction

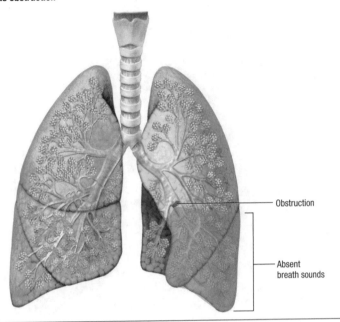

Obstruction

Absent
breath sounds

If a mainstem bronchus is obstructed, breath sounds are absent
throughout the entire affected lung. (See *Mainstem bronchus
obstruction*, page 150.)

 ALERT *Aspirated foreign bodies are more likely to lodge in
the right mainstem bronchus because it provides a more
direct vertical passage than the left. For the same reason,
endotracheal tubes are commonly misplaced in the right mainstem
bronchus. If breath sounds are absent throughout the left lung
field after intubation, the endotracheal tube must be repositioned.*

 ALERT *When a patient has aspirated a foreign body and
continues to cough, don't intervene—allow the patient to
cough up the foreign body, if possible.*

Pneumothorax
A pneumothorax is the accumulation of air in the normally airless
pleural space because of a tear in either the visceral or parietal
pleura. Breath sounds heard over a pneumothorax are significantly diminished or absent because of acoustic mismatching of
the air-filled lung and the collection of air in the pleural space.
(◆Sound 72)
The degree of change in breath sounds depends on the size
of the pneumothorax. A small pneumothorax may not alter the
breath sound intensity enough to be heard during auscultation;
it may, however, be apparent on a chest X-ray. A large pneumothorax significantly diminishes breath sounds or permits no

Mainstem bronchus obstruction

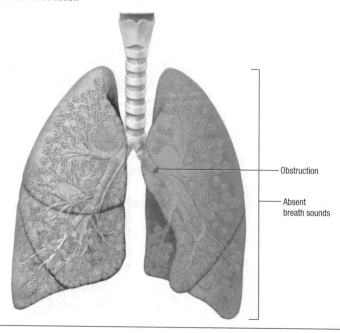

Obstruction

Absent
breath sounds

sound transmission, causing absent breath sounds. Typical pneumothorax characteristics include sharp, stabbing chest pain; dyspnea; absent breath sounds; inaudible egophony, bronchophony, and whispered pectoriloquy; and increased resonance during percussion.

ALERT *A pneumothorax that continues to increase in size may be life-threatening, particularly if the patient is being ventilated mechanically. If the increasing intrapleural air isn't evacuated immediately, intrathoracic pressure may increase, causing decreased cardiac output, hypotension, and eventual death.*

Sound characteristics
Diminished or absent breath sounds resulting from a pneumothorax can occur anywhere over the anterior, posterior, and lateral chest wall surfaces, depending on the location and size of the pneumothorax.

In a patient with a pneumothorax in the left lateral lung field—the area over the fourth, fifth, sixth, and seventh intercostal spaces between the anterior and posterior axillary folds—normal breath sounds are heard on the contralateral side over healthy lung tissue (♦**Sound 73**), and breath sounds are absent over the pneumothorax. (♦**Sound 74**) If diminished breath sounds are heard, they have a low pitch that's heard using either the bell or diaphragm of the stethoscope.

Pneumothorax affecting left lateral lung field

Affected lung area

Pleural effusion

In pleural effusion, fluid accumulates in the pleural space, impairing the transmission of normal breath sounds. Because of the acoustical mismatch, breath sounds are diminished or absent. **(♦Sound 75)**

A large pleural effusion compresses adjacent lung tissue, causing atelectasis; the percussion tone is dull. Egophony, bronchophony, and whispered pectoriloquy caused by the atelectasis may be audible at the upper border of the pleural effusion. Occasionally, loud bronchial breath sounds may have sufficient intensity to be transmitted through a small pleural effusion.

Sound characteristics

Diminished or absent breath sounds resulting from a pleural effusion may occur anywhere over the anterior, posterior, or lateral chest wall surfaces, depending on the location of the pleural effusion.

In a patient with a pleural effusion in the right posterior lower lung field, diminished breath sounds are heard over the eighth, ninth, and tenth intercostal spaces from the vertebral line to just right of the midscapular line and normal breath sounds are heard on the contralateral side over healthy lung tissue. **(♦Sound 76)** The diminished breath sounds have a low pitch that can be heard using either the bell or diaphragm of the stethoscope. **(♦Sound 77)**

Pleural effusion affecting right lower lobe

Affected lung area

Posterior auscultatory sites

ALERT *If the pleural effusion is large, diminished or absent sounds can be heard over the lower right anterior and lateral chest wall surfaces as well. Monitor the patient for respiratory distress, and prepare for chest tube insertion, if necessary.*

Hyperinflated lungs

Hyperinflated lungs, typical of patients with chronic obstructive pulmonary disease (COPD) or severe asthma, impede breath sound transmission in the following way: Premature dynamic compression of the large central airways and the loss of elastic tension in the lung tissue limit airflow during expiration. Increased intrinsic airway resistance may also be present. Increased amounts of air trapped in the lungs change the acoustical qualities of the sound transmitted, creating a mismatch between the pleurae and chest wall, and the hyperinflated lung tissue. Consequently, the breath sounds are diminished. (♦**Sound 78**)

The intensity of those breath sounds is directly related to the severity of the COPD. For example, patients with marked hyperinflation typically have an increased anterior-to-posterior thoracic diameter and a flattened and immobile diaphragm. Breath sounds aren't as loud as usual because of the increased mismatch produced by trapped air and because less air is being moved during each respiratory cycle. Other signs and symptoms of COPD include a hyperresonant percussion note, dyspnea (a primary sign of severe COPD), prolonged expiratory phase, and inaudible egophony, bronchophony, and whispered pectoriloquy.

ALERT *If a patient with COPD has breath sounds that have progressed from diminished to absent, prepare for endotracheal intubation and mechanical ventilation.*

Sound characteristics

Diminished or absent breath sounds associated with COPD are heard over the anterior, posterior, and lateral chest wall surfaces. If breath sounds are audible, they're soft in intensity and they have a low pitch that's heard best using the diaphragm of the stethoscope. These sounds are heard throughout inspiration and expiration. (♦**Sound 78**)

Obesity

Breath sounds are normally attenuated and filtered at the pleural surface. In an obese person, a thickened chest wall increases the distance between lung tissue and the chest wall surface, creating an impedance mismatch. This filters breath sounds as they're transmitted from the pleurae to the chest wall surface. (♦**Sound 79**)

Sound characteristics

Diminished breath sounds are heard over the anterior, posterior, and lateral chest wall surfaces. The location of fat pads determines where the breath sounds are most difficult to hear. For best results when auscultating an obese patient's lungs, ask him to sit up. Then ask him to take deep breaths through an open mouth while you listen.

Positive end-expiratory pressure

Adding PEEP during mechanical ventilation of an intubated patient can diminish breath sounds in the following way: PEEP increases functional residual capacity (FRC), the amount of air remaining in the airways at the end of normal expiration. Increasing FRC hyperinflates the lungs.

Sound characteristics

Diminished breath sounds occur because increased amounts of air in the small airways and alveoli change the acoustical qualities of the sound transmitted through the chest wall, creating a mismatch between the pleurae and chest wall, and the hyperinflated lung. (♦Sound 80)

♦♦♦POSTTEST

1. What causes diminished or absent breath sounds?
2. Explain why shallow breathing results in diminished breath sounds.
3. Describe the changes in airflow distal to an obstruction.
4. Why does a pneumothorax cause diminished or absent breath sounds?
5. Describe the breath sound characteristics associated with a large pneumothorax.
6. Describe the breath sound characteristics associated with a pleural effusion.
7. Why do hyperinflated lungs cause diminished or absent breath sounds?
8. Describe the breath sound characteristics associated with chronic obstructive pulmonary disease.
9. How does obesity change the characteristics of normal breath sounds?
10. Explain the effects of PEEP on breath sounds.

Other abnormal breath sounds

18 Classifying adventitious sounds

PRETEST ◆◆◆

1. Name the two types of adventitious sounds.
2. Describe the difference between fine and coarse crackles.
3. Describe the difference between wheezes and low-pitched wheezes.

CONFUSION OVER TERMINOLOGY

The methods of classifying adventitious sounds have changed repeatedly over the years, resulting in continuing confusion in the literature and in the clinical setting. The familiar terms used by Laënnec were replaced by terms that later physicians thought were more aesthetic or clearer. For example, the term *rhonchus* was substituted for *rale* because the latter was associated with the "death rattle" sound. Later, attempts were made to classify adventitious sounds on the basis of their acoustic qualities or their similarities to musical tones.

CURRENT CLASSIFICATION SYSTEM

In 1977, the American Thoracic Society adopted a system of classifying adventitious sounds on the basis of acoustical qualities, timing, and frequency waveforms. This system divides adventitious sounds into two classifications: crackles and wheezes. These two classifications are further subdivided into two categories: discontinuous and continuous.

Discontinuous, explosive sounds that are loud and low-pitched are called *coarse crackles*. **(◆Sound 81)** Previously, these sounds were called *rales* or *coarse rales*.

Discontinuous, explosive sounds that are shorter in duration, soft and higher in pitch, and less intense than coarse crackles are called *fine crackles*. **(◆Sound 82)** Previously, these sounds were called *fine rales* or *crepitations*.

Continuous sounds that are high-pitched and have a hissing sound are called *wheezes*. Wheezes commonly have a musical quality. **(◆Sound 83)** Previously, these sounds were called *sibilant rales* or *sibilant rhonchi*.

Continuous sounds that are low-pitched and commonly resemble snoring are called *low-pitched wheezes*. **(◆Sound 84)** Previously, these sounds were called *sonorous rales* or *sonorous rhonchi*.

It should be noted that the term *rhonchi* is still commonly used in the clinical setting, rather than *low-pitched wheezes*. Rhonchus is used to describe a rough, rumbling low-pitched sound that is heard primarily on expiration, although, at times, rhonchi may also be heard with inspiration. Rhonchi are generally caused by fluid or secretions partially blocking the large airways and typically change in sound, or disappear, with coughing.

◀◀◀ POSTTEST

1. What are the two classifications of adventitious sounds?
2. Describe coarse crackles.
3. Describe fine crackles.
4. Describe wheezes.
5. Describe low-pitched wheezes.

19 Adventitious sounds: crackles

PRETEST ▸▸▸

1. What causes crackles?
2. What is the difference between coarse and fine crackles?
3. Describe the characteristics of late inspiratory crackles.
4. Describe the characteristics of early inspiratory and expiratory crackles.
5. Describe the characteristics of pleural crackles.

SOUND PRODUCTION

Crackles, formerly known as rales, are discontinuous, intermittent, nonmusical sounds that are described according to their timing and duration within the respiratory phase, intensity, pitch, and location. These short, explosive or popping sounds are heard primarily through the chest wall with a stethoscope, but they may also be heard at the mouth with or without a stethoscope. Crackles are characterized as fine or coarse. Fine crackles have a soft, high-pitched, very brief nature and coarse crackles are louder, lower in pitch, and are brief but slightly longer than the fine ones. The characteristics of crackles change, depending on the underlying cause. Two different mechanisms are thought to generate crackles: air bubbling through secretions and the sudden, explosive opening of airways.

Air bubbling through secretions

Air bubbling through secretions in the airways is widely accepted as one way crackles are produced. According to Dr. Paul Forgacs, this explanation is probably true when the trachea and mainstem bronchi are full of sputum, as commonly occurs with severe pulmonary edema and chronic bronchitis. However, Forgacs argues that the air bubbling theory doesn't explain why crackles are heard mainly during inspiration and why they're heard over diseased lungs when sputum is usually absent. Further, in the smaller airways, airflow resistance—produced by the surface tension and viscosity of secretions—is too high to be overcome by the air pressure gradients that are present in healthy lungs during inspiration and expiration. Thus, another mechanism must explain how crackles are produced in the smaller airways.

Sudden, explosive opening of airways

At the end of expiration, peripheral airways in the lung bases close. At the beginning of inspiration, these peripheral airways remain closed, and inspired air flows to each lung apex first. The airways that are distal to the closed peripheral airways remain underexpanded until airway pressures and external forces, such as diaphragmatic movement and rib cage expansion, snap the airways open. The sudden opening of multiple collapsed peripheral airways and the associated explosive changes in air pressures are thought to produce the crackles heard over the lung bases in a healthy person who inhales deeply after a maximum exhalation. This mechanism is also thought to be responsible for the crackles heard in patients with atelectasis and interstitial lung disease.

Crackles are acoustic alterations that follow abrupt equalization of pressures or a change in elasticity resulting from the sudden opening of abnormally closed airways. Crackles are characterized by a repetitive rhythm and loudness. These characteristics suggest that the airways open in the same sequence, at the same point in the respiratory cycle, and at the same approximate lung volumes. Crackles may be present in the lung bases of older individuals and occasionally in other healthy individuals. These crackles clear with coughing and have no pathological significance.

 AGE ISSUE *Crackles aren't usually heard in infants; however, if present, they could indicate respiratory tract infection.*

DOCUMENTATION

The timing of crackles is described as early inspiration, midinspiration, or late inspiration or early expiration, midexpiration, or late expiration. The duration, indicating the length of time that the crackles can be heard during inspiration or expiration, varies. Sound intensity is described as soft, intermediate, loud, or very loud. Pitch is considered high or low. The density of crackles in the thoracic region is described as diffuse or scanty.

LATE INSPIRATORY CRACKLES

Late inspiratory crackles are high-pitched, explosive sounds of variable intensity and density. These are heard mostly over dependent or poorly ventilated lung regions.

Related conditions
Conditions associated with late inspiratory crackles include atelectasis, resolving lobar pneumonia, interstitial fibrosis, and left-sided heart failure.

Atelectasis
Atelectasis, the incomplete expansion of a lung area, is seen in postoperative and immobile patients and in patients with impaired diaphragmatic function. Resorption of alveolar air occurs secondary to prolonged hypoventilation, gravitational forces that close airways and deflate the lung bases, obstruction from secretions, and mucus plugging the airways. The result is poor ventilation

Late inspiratory crackles heard over lower lobes

Affected lung area

Posterior auscultatory sites

in the affected areas and possible collapse of segmental or lobar bronchi. If small peripheral airways are involved, clinical findings may not be detectable. However, if a larger airway is involved, the clinical findings of decreased chest wall movement, a dull percussion note, and bronchial breath sounds are easily noted. The transmission of vocal sounds, such as egophony, bronchophony, and whispered pectoriloquy, suggests atelectasis.

Crackles associated with atelectasis are produced by the sudden opening of collapsed small airways and adjoining alveoli. These crackles are high-pitched, explosive sounds heard late in inspiration. (**♦Sound 85**)

AGE ISSUE *Premature infants may develop atelectasis secondary to a surfactant deficiency. Older adults on prolonged bed rest are especially susceptible to atelectasis due to changes in their musculoskeletal systems (such as kyphosis, which decreases lung expansion) and decreased respiratory and expiratory forces.*

Sound characteristics

In a postoperative patient who hasn't been coughing and deep breathing adequately, late inspiratory crackles are heard over the posterior bases of both lungs. This area is located between the eighth and tenth intercostal spaces from the left posterior axillary line to the right posterior axillary line. The crackles begin late in inspiration and become more profuse toward the end of inspiration. They vary in intensity but are high-pitched. (**♦Sound 85**)

Because crackles associated with atelectasis are poorly transmitted to the chest wall surface, their intensity and density change when the stethoscope is moved only a short distance. Crackles are not audible at the mouth. The patient's position affects the detection of crackles. For example, in an immobile patient, profuse

Late inspiratory crackles heard over right middle lobe

Affected lung area

Anterior auscultatory sites

crackles are heard in the dependent lung regions, but crackles are absent or scanty in the nondependent lung regions. Also, crackles associated with atelectasis may clear somewhat with coughing.

Lobar pneumonia

In patients with resolving lobar pneumonia, crackles can be auscultated over lung areas where many alveoli are still filled with exudate, but the surrounding alveoli are aerated and have higher-than-normal ventilation. A large increase in air pressure gradients in the airways reaching these unaerated alveoli generates crackles as the airways are snapped open during late inspiration. These crackles have a sound similar to that of late inspiratory crackles heard over atelectatic areas, but are not affected by coughing or position changes. **(♦Sound 86)**

AGE ISSUE *Older adults are at greater risk for developing pneumonia because their weakened chest muscles reduce their ability to clear secretions. Bacterial pneumonia is the most common type found in older adults; viral pneumonia, the second most common. Aspiration pneumonia occurs from impaired swallowing ability and a diminished gag reflex due to prolonged illness or a neurological disorder, such as stroke.*

Sound characteristics

In a patient with right middle lobe pneumonia, late inspiratory crackles are heard over the right anterior chest wall surface between the third and fifth intercostal spaces. It is imperative to auscultate the right lateral lobe during examination. Crackles begin late in inspiration and become more profuse toward the end of inspiration. They begin late in inspiration and become more profuse toward the end of inspiration. These crackles are typically high-pitched. **(♦Sound 86)**

Lung area where right and left lateral late inspiratory crackles are heard

Interstitial fibrosis

Diffuse interstitial fibrosis impairs or destroys alveoli by filling them with abnormal cells or by scarring the lung tissue. Unaffected alveoli are usually hyperaerated. The lungs become stiff and nonelastic and become more difficult to inflate; airflow volumes usually decrease. Theoretically, the delayed opening of small airways during inspiration causes alveolar pressures in the affected lung tissue to fall more significantly than in healthy alveoli. This fall in alveolar pressures leads to an increased pressure gradient that generates repetitive fine, late inspiratory crackles. (**♦Sound 87**) Coughing doesn't affect the profusion of crackles.

With mild interstitial fibrosis, crackles are auscultated at the end of inspiration over dependent lung regions—usually over the lateral lung bases when the patient is seated upright. Crackles can disappear if the patient inhales deeply, holds his breath, or leans forward. However, they usually recur when the patient returns to the upright position.

As interstitial fibrosis worsens, crackles are heard bilaterally over the posterior lung bases and spread upward toward the apices. In later stages of the disease, crackles are not affected by position changes and may be heard throughout inspiration.

Either interstitial fibrosis or interstitial pneumonitis is associated with interstitial and alveolar infiltrates. Patients with a significant amount of lung involvement have dyspnea and a cough. Interstitial fibrosis may be caused by inhalation of heavy metals, the antibiotic nitrofurantoin, some chemotherapeutic agents, or prolonged inhalation of high concentrations of oxygen. In most cases, however, the cause is unknown.

Crackles heard in patients with known exposure to asbestos are thought to be an early sign of asbestosis, a lung disease characterized by pulmonary inflammation and fibrosis. The profusion of crackles increases in proportion to the amount of exposure to asbestos.

Pulmonary sarcoidosis, a noncaseating granulomatous disease of unknown cause that occurs in the lungs and other organs, may progress to interstitial fibrosis, resulting in restrictive lung disease. The connective tissue disorders such as rheumatoid arthritis and scleroderma are also associated with diffuse interstitial fibrosis.

Sound characteristics

Crackles associated with interstitial fibrosis caused by early asbestosis are initially heard in the midaxillary area over the lateral lung bases, the area over the seventh and eighth intercostal spaces. As the disease progresses, they may be heard over the posterior bases and may spread toward the apices and are heard during late inspiration. These crackles have a fine intensity and a short, discontinuous duration. These crackles have a high pitch that is appreciated using the diaphragm of the stethoscope. (**♦Sound 87**)

Late inspiratory crackles heard over posterior lung bases

Affected lung area

Posterior auscultatory sites

Left-sided heart failure

Left-sided heart failure leads to fluid accumulation in the lung interstitium. Crackles are produced by the rapid equalization of pressures associated with the delayed opening of airways narrowed by pulmonary edema. They're commonly auscultated over the posterior lung bases in the early stages of pulmonary edema. Profuse and high-pitched **(♦Sound 88)**, these crackles are inaudible at the mouth. Common signs and symptoms of left-sided heart failure include dyspnea, orthopnea, hypoxia, cough, cyanosis or pallor, arrhythmias, and pulsus alternans. If pulmonary edema worsens, the airways are flooded with fluids. This results in severe hypoxia and low-pitched inspiratory and expiratory crackles that may be audible at the mouth and over the entire chest wall surface.

 AUSCULTATION TIP *In the patient with heart failure, auscultate the lung bases first because crackles may not be audible after continued deep breaths.*

Sound characteristics

Crackles associated with early left-sided heart failure and pulmonary edema are heard bilaterally over the posterior lung bases, the area over the eighth, ninth, and tenth intercostal spaces. As pulmonary edema worsens, the crackles become more profuse and may be heard throughout the chest during late inspiration; the duration varies with the degree of failure. Their intensity is fine in the early stages of left-sided heart failure but changes to a loud rattling sound as the patient's condition worsens. Crackles having a low pitch are appreciated using either the bell or the diaphragm of the stethoscope. **(♦Sound 88)**

EARLY INSPIRATORY AND EXPIRATORY CRACKLES

Coarse crackles occur during early inspiration and during expiration. They're common in diffuse airway obstruction and may be heard over any chest wall area. Coarse crackles have a lower pitch than fine crackles and, although these are usually loud and may disappear after a cough, these are unaffected by the patient's position.

Coarse crackles typically are heard in an irregular rhythm that may be interrupted by short sequences of evenly spaced crackles having the same intensity. These crackles may arise from intermittent closure of large bronchi and the corresponding flow of a bolus of air through the obstructed area.

Related conditions

Crackles are also associated with chronic bronchitis and bronchiectasis.

Chronic bronchitis

Early inspiratory crackles are associated with excessive mucus production in patients with chronic bronchitis. The proliferation and hypertrophy of mucous glands within the airways are caused by chronic exposure to airway irritants, such as cigarette smoke (the most common) and air pollution. Coughing, sputum production, and repeated respiratory tract infections are common in patients with chronic bronchitis. Chronic bronchitis can lead to chronic obstructive pulmonary disease. (♦Sound 89)

Sound characteristics

In patients with chronic bronchitis, crackles are heard early in inspiration, over all chest wall surfaces, and at the mouth. These crackles are low-pitched, scanty, and are not affected by the patient's position. (♦Sound 89)

Bronchiectasis

Bronchiectasis, irreversible dilation of the bronchi in selected lung segments, is characterized by chronic and copious production of yellow or green sputum and by fibrotic or atelectatic lung tissue surrounding the affected airways. Evidence of old inflammatory changes in the patient's lungs is usually noted on the chest X-ray.

Causes of bronchiectasis include foreign body obstruction, tumor, viral or bacterial pneumonia (particularly repeated childhood pneumonias), chronic inflammatory or fibrotic lung disease, and tuberculosis. (♦Sound 90)

Auscultatory sites for profuse early-to-midinspiratory crackles

Anterior view

Posterior view

Sound characteristics

In patients with left midlung and lower lung area bronchiectasis, crackles are heard over the patient's anterior, posterior, and left lateral chest wall surfaces. The anterior area is located over the fourth, fifth, and sixth intercostal spaces, and the posterior area is located over the seventh, eighth, ninth, and tenth intercostal spaces. In patients with bronchiectasis, crackles tend to be profuse, low-pitched, heard during early or midinspiration, and coarser than those associated with chronic bronchitis. Coughing may decrease the number of crackles heard, but changes in the patient's position do not affect them. (◆**Sound 90**)

Lung area where profuse early-to-midinspiratory crackles are heard

Auscultatory site for pleural crackles heard over right midlung

Anterior view

Lung area where right midlung pleural crackles are heard

PLEURAL CRACKLES

When the visceral and parietal pleural surfaces are damaged by fibrin deposits or inflammatory or neoplastic cells, they lose their ability to glide silently over each other during breathing; movements become jerky and periodically delayed. This motion produces loud, grating crackles known as *pleural crackles* or *pleural friction rub*. (♦**Sound 91)** These crackles may be present during the inspiratory and expiratory phases of the respiratory cycle, or they may be confined only to inspiration. Pleural crackles disappear if fluid accumulates between the pleurae.

Pleural crackles are usually associated with sharp pain during inspiration, which may cause the patient to spontaneously splint the affected side to minimize muscle movement and chest expansion. Asymmetrical chest wall movement in the patient may be palpable, and a rapid, shallow-breathing pattern may also be present.

AGE ISSUE *If a child has grunting respirations, reports chest pain, or protects his chest by holding it or lying on one side, auscultate for pleural crackles, an early sign of pleurisy.*

Sound characteristics

Pleural crackles are heard on the chest wall over the affected area. When pleural crackles are heard over the patient's right midlung—the area over the fifth and sixth intercostal spaces between the right midclavicular and right midaxillary lines—their intensity is loud and they have a coarse, grating quality and a low pitch. (♦**Sound 91)** Their duration is discontinuous. Pleural crackles may be heard during inspiration only or during both the inspiratory and expiratory phases of the respiratory cycle.

AUSCULTATION TIP *To distinguish between a pleural friction rub and a pericardial friction rub, have the patient hold his breath; if the rub continues, it's a pericardial friction rub.*

◀◀◀ POSTTEST

1. What are the characteristics of crackles?
2. Name the four conditions associated with late inspiratory crackles.
3. Describe the characteristics of crackles associated with atelectasis.
4. Describe the characteristics of crackles associated with resolving lobar pneumonia.
5. How does interstitial fibrosis cause crackles?
6. How are crackles generated in the patient with left-sided heart failure?
7. Describe the characteristics of coarse crackles.
8. Explain how early inspiratory crackles arise in the patient with chronic bronchitis.
9. Describe the characteristics of crackles associated with bronchiectasis.
10. Differentiate the characteristics of pleural crackles from other crackles.

PRETEST ▸▸▸

1. Describe the mechanism that produces wheezing?
2. What conditions are associated with wheezes?
3. Describe the following types of wheezes: expiratory polyphonic, fixed monophonic, sequential inspiratory, and random monophonic.
4. What type of wheeze is associated with asthma?
5. Widespread airflow obstruction causes what type of wheezing?
6. Describe stridor.

Airflow pattern in narrowed bronchus

1. Airway wall
2. Narrowed bronchus

Oscillations of narrowed bronchus

1. Airway wall
2. Narrowed bronchus

SOUND PRODUCTION

Wheezes—which are associated with such conditions as bronchospasm, airway thickening caused by mucosal swelling or muscle hypertrophy, inhalation of a foreign body, tumor, secretions, and dynamic airway compression—are musical sounds generated by air passing through a bronchus so narrowed as to be almost closed. The bronchus walls oscillate between closed and barely open positions; these oscillations generate audible sounds.

Wheezes are musical, relatively high-pitched, continuous sounds with frequencies of ≥400 Hz and a duration of ≥250 milliseconds. Their duration is long enough to carry an audible pitch similar to a musical tone that may often sound like hissing. Wheezes are described by their timing within the respiratory cycle; they may be heard during inspiration or expiration or continuously throughout the respiratory cycle. Wheezes can be further described as localized or diffuse, episodic or chronic.

Frequency

A wheeze's pitch is determined by the emitted sound's frequency, which can vary widely over a five-octave range. These differences in frequency are attributed to the airway size and elasticity and to airflow rates through the narrowed bronchus. Theoretically, large, flabby, narrowed airways generate low-pitched sounds; stiff, narrowed airways generate high-pitched sounds. Pitch does not correlate to airway length, width, or to air density.

Wheezes of different pitches may occur simultaneously or may overlap, and the pitch of a single wheeze may change during inspiration and expiration. *Monophonic wheezes* produce single musical notes that may vary in duration and may overlap. *Polyphonic wheezes* combine several distinct musical tones.

Transmission

Wheezes are transmitted better through airways than through lung tissue, which absorbs high-frequency sounds. Wheezes that sound louder over central airways than over peripheral lung tissue may be sounds transmitted through the central airways but are not produced by them. Wheezes heard at the mouth in severe airway obstruction may not be audible during auscultation of the chest wall surfaces.

 ALERT *Be alert for impending respiratory failure if wheezes are audible at the mouth and breath sounds are diminished or absent.*

EXPIRATORY POLYPHONIC WHEEZES

Polyphonic wheezes are thought to be caused by the dynamic compression of large airways during expiration. In healthy individuals, polyphonic wheezes can sometimes be auscultated during a maximal forced expiration when the dynamic compression occurs simultaneously in all airways. No regional variations exist in airway resistance or in lung compliance; consequently, polyphonic wheezes are heard throughout the lungs during expiration.

Polyphonic wheezes are loud, musical, and widely transmitted; when heard during regular breathing, they indicate widespread airflow obstruction.

In patients with widespread airflow obstruction (as in asthma, chronic obstructive pulmonary disease, chronic bronchitis), elastic recoil properties, peripheral airway resistance, and airway mechanics are altered throughout both lungs. Together, these abnormal changes affect the timing of dynamic airway compression within the bronchi, which alters normal sound production. For example, during sequential forceful expirations, the central bronchi are compressed first when elastic recoil of the airways is low or when peripheral airway resistance is high. This compression produces a series of sounds, beginning with a monophonic wheeze and quickly followed by bitonal sounds. Soon, the full complement of sounds that make up polyphonic wheezes are audible through the stethoscope. These multiple musical tones begin simultaneously and maintain a constant pitch that rises sharply at the end of expiration. **(♦Sound 92)**

Sound characteristics

Expiratory polyphonic wheezes are usually heard over the anterior, posterior, and lateral chest wall surfaces during expiration. Their intensity is usually described as loud and musical, and their duration is continuous. They have a high pitch that is heard best using the diaphragm of the stethoscope. **(♦Sound 93)**

Auscultatory sites for fixed monophonic wheezes

Anterior view

Posterior view

Lung area where fixed monophonic wheezes are heard

Partially obstructed lobar bronchus

FIXED MONOPHONIC WHEEZES

Fixed monophonic wheezes, which have a constant pitch and a single musical tone, are generated by the oscillations of a large, partially obstructed bronchus. The obstruction may be caused by a tumor, a foreign body, bronchial stenosis, or an intrabronchial granuloma; each of these conditions narrows the airway but doesn't slow airflow. Fixed monophonic wheezes are low-pitched and are transmitted throughout the lungs. (◆**Sound 94**)

In a patient with bronchial stenosis, the pitch of inspiratory and expiratory monophonic wheezes varies, depending on airway rigidity. Monophonic wheezes may disappear when the patient is in a supine position or turns from side to side and may clear slightly following coughing.

Lung area where sequential inspiratory wheezes are heard

Auscultatory sites for sequential inspiratory wheezes

Posterior view

Sound characteristics

In a patient with a partially obstructed right lobar bronchus, fixed monophonic wheezes are heard over the anterior, posterior, and right lateral chest wall surfaces. The anterior area is located over the third, fourth, fifth, and sixth intercostal spaces; the posterior area is located over the fifth, sixth, seventh, eighth, ninth, and tenth intercostal spaces. Fixed monophonic wheezes are usually loud, and their duration is continuous. They may be heard during inspiration, expiration, or throughout the respiratory cycle. They have a low pitch that is heard best using the diaphragm of the stethoscope. (♦**Sound 94**)

SEQUENTIAL INSPIRATORY WHEEZES

Sequential inspiratory wheezes are sometimes heard over the lung bases in patients with interstitial fibrosis, asbestosis, or fibrosing or extrinsic allergic alveolitis. These monophonic wheezes are generated by airways that open late in inspiration in unaerated lung regions. The rapid inflow of air precipitates airway wall vibrations, generating sequential inspiratory wheezes.

A single, short inspiratory wheeze or a brief sequence of monophonic inspiratory wheezes with different pitches may be heard along with the crackles normally associated with interstitial fibrosis. (◆**Sound 94**)

Sound characteristics
Sequential inspiratory wheezes are usually heard over the lateral and posterior lung bases. On the posterior chest wall surface, this area is located over the eighth, ninth, and tenth intercostal spaces; on the lateral chest wall surfaces, it is located over the seventh and eighth intercostal spaces. Sequential inspiratory wheezes have a loud intensity and a continuous duration. They occur throughout inspiration but are more predominant in late inspiration. They have a high pitch that is heard best using the diaphragm of the stethoscope. (◆**Sound 94**)

RANDOM MONOPHONIC WHEEZES

Airways narrowed by bronchospasm or mucosal swelling produce single or multiple monophonic wheezes that may occur during inspiration, expiration, or throughout the respiratory cycle. Multiple wheezes can occur randomly and vary in duration. Random monophonic wheezes produced in the large central airways are loud and widely transmitted throughout the lung; they can be heard at a distance from the mouth. (◆**Sound 95**) In contrast, random monophonic wheezes produced in the peripheral airways are weaker and are filtered through transmission to the chest wall; these sounds are audible only over the chest wall.

Random monophonic wheezes are typically heard in patients with severe status asthmaticus. In such patients, airway resistance is high; dynamic airway compression moves from the central airways toward the smaller peripheral airways, where the airflow rate is too low to produce airway wall vibrations or sounds.

The progressive airway obstruction that occurs in patients with status asthmaticus can cause a dynamic pattern of wheezing. First, monophonic wheezes are heard only during expiration. They are heard throughout the respiratory cycle. Monophonic wheezes may also be heard at the mouth because the high-frequency sounds are transmitted through larger airways.

ALERT *Status asthmaticus is a life-threatening condition. As the severity of the condition worsens, all wheezes heard over the chest wall surfaces disappear. The combination of air trapping and severe airway narrowing causes the site of dynamic airway compression to move toward the lung periphery; this phenomenon is called a silent chest. Silent chest is commonly accompanied by hypercapnia (increased carbon dioxide levels in the blood) and acidosis; both conditions may be fatal.*

Sound characteristics

Random monophonic wheezes are usually heard over the anterior, posterior, and lateral chest wall surfaces. They are usually loud, and their duration is continuous. These wheezes occur throughout the respiratory cycle, and expiration is frequently prolonged. They have a high pitch that is heard best using the diaphragm of the stethoscope.

STRIDOR

Stridor is a loud musical sound that can be heard at a distance from the patient, usually without a stethoscope. Laryngeal spasm and mucosal swelling cause contraction of the vocal cords and airway constriction, causing stridor. The loud monophonic wheeze of stridor is typically heard during inspiration, but it also may be heard throughout the respiratory cycle as airway constriction increases. Its intensity distinguishes it from other monophonic wheezes. (**♦Sound 96**) Stridor is most commonly associated with severe upper respiratory infections, whooping cough, laryngeal tumors, tracheal stenosis, and aspiration of a foreign object. Conscious individuals with stridor will assume a high-Fowler's position as they attempt to ventilate.

 ALERT *Children with acute epiglottitis have stridor that worsens when in the supine position. During throat examination, trained personnel, such as an anesthesiologist, should be present to secure an emergency airway. Special equipment, such as a laryngoscope and an endotracheal tube, should be available because a tongue blade can cause sudden, complete airway obstruction.*

Sound characteristics

Severe stridor is heard without a stethoscope; however, in a patient with a less-pronounced laryngeal spasm, stridor may be heard by auscultating over the larynx. Stridor is loud and has a continuous duration. It may be heard during inspiration or throughout the respiratory cycle. Its high pitch resembles a crowing sound. (**♦Sound 96**)

 ALERT *If the patient with stridor is drooling, the epiglottis may be severely swollen. Do not examine the mouth. Any stimulus could worsen the airway occlusion. Immediate medical intervention is necessary. The patient may require emergency intubation or tracheotomy.*

◀◀◀ POSTTEST

1. Define the term *wheezes*.
2. What are the characteristics of wheezes?
3. Name the five conditions associated with wheezes.
4. Describe the characteristics of expiratory polyphonic wheezes.
5. How are fixed monophonic wheezes generated?
6. What conditions are associated with sequential inspiratory wheezes?
7. How are sequential inspiratory wheezes generated?
8. How are random monophonic wheezes generated?
9. How can the characteristics of random monophonic wheezes be expected to change as asthma worsens?
10. Describe stridor.

**Auscultation findings for
common disorders**

**Assessment flowcharts for
common auscultation findings**

**English-Spanish phrases used in cardiac
and respiratory assessment**

Posttest answers

Selected readings

Additional web site

Glossary

Index

Auscultation findings for common disorders

The following is a compilation of various cardiac and pulmonary disorders along with associated auscultation findings. The patient may not present with every assessment finding listed for each disorder.

Disorder	Abnormal breath sounds	Abnormal heart sounds
Aortic prosthetic valve		• Systolic murmur • Aortic opening click • Aortic closing click • Interval between aortic closing click and P_2 that widens during inspiration
Aortic regurgitation		• Early diastolic murmur often with midsystolic murmur • "Cooing dove" or "musical" diastolic murmur signifies rupture or retroversion of an aortic cusp • Diminished A_2 • Early ejection click • Paradoxical S_2 split • S_3 and S_4 • Soft S_1
Aortic valvular stenosis	• Inspiratory and expiratory crackles over the posterior lung bases associated with heart failure	• Midsystolic murmur that decreases with Valsalva maneuver • Paradoxical S_2 split • Delayed A_2 and shortened A_2-P_2 interval • Aortic ejection sound radiates widely to neck and along great vessels • Systolic ejection sound if not severely stenotic
Asbestosis	• High-pitched crackles heard at the end of inspiration • Crackles throughout entire inspiratory phase (with advanced disease) • Pleural friction rub	Only when severe: • Paradoxical S_2 split • Right ventricular heave

Disorder	Abnormal breath sounds	Abnormal heart sounds
Asthma	▪ Diminished breath sounds ▪ Musical, high-pitched expiratory polyphonic wheezes ▪ With status asthmaticus, loud and continuous random monophonic wheezes heard, along with prolonged expiration and possible silent chest if severe	
Atelectasis	▪ High-pitched, hollow, tubular bronchial breath sounds, crackles, wheezes ▪ Fine, high-pitched late inspiratory crackles ▪ Diminished breath sounds over affected area ▪ Bronchophony ▪ Egophony ▪ Whispered pectoriloquy ▪ I:E ratio: I > E over empty lung field	
Atrial septal defect		▪ Wide, fixed S_2 split ▪ Pulmonic ejection sound ▪ Tricuspid component louder than mitral component
Bronchial stenosis	▪ Loud, continuous, low-pitched, fixed, monophonic wheezes that may disappear when in supine position or turning side to side	
Bronchiectasis	▪ Profuse, low-pitched crackles heard during midinspiration ▪ Scattered wheezing	
Chronic bronchitis	▪ Scanty, low-pitched, early inspiratory crackles not affected by patient's position ▪ Loud, musical, high-pitched, expiratory polyphonic wheezes	

(*continued*)

Disorder	Abnormal breath sounds	Abnormal heart sounds
Chronic obstructive pulmonary disease	▪ Diminished, low-pitched breath sounds ▪ Sonorous and/or sibilant wheezes ▪ Inaudible bronchophony, egophony, and whispered pectoriloquy ▪ Prolonged expiration ▪ Fine inspiratory crackles	▪ Paradoxical S_2 split ▪ Right ventricular heave
Fibrosing alveolitis	▪ Loud, continuous, high-pitched, sequential wheezes	
Hypertrophic obstructive cardiomyopathy	▪ Inspiratory and expiratory crackles over the posterior lung bases associated with heart failure	▪ Midsystolic murmur that becomes louder with Valsalva maneuver ▪ Paradoxical S_2 split ▪ S_3 and S_4
Interstitial pulmonary fibrosis	▪ Late inspiratory fine crackles not affected by coughing but may disappear with position change, deep inhalation, or holding of breath ▪ High-pitched bronchial or bronchovesicular breath sounds heard over lower lung regions that are audible through inspiration and expiration ▪ Loud, high-pitched sequential wheezes of continuous duration ▪ Whispered pectoriloquy	
Laryngeal spasm	▪ Stridor heard during inspiration	
Malfunctioning aortic prosthetic valve	▪ Inspiratory and expiratory crackles over the posterior lung bases associated with heart failure	▪ Long systolic ejection murmur ▪ Absent or softened aortic opening click ▪ Absent or diminished aortic closing click ▪ Diastolic murmur
Malfunctioning mitral prosthetic valve	▪ Inspiratory and expiratory crackles over the posterior lung bases associated with heart failure	▪ Holosystolic murmur ▪ New diastolic murmur or change in intensity or duration of existing one ▪ Diastolic rumble ▪ Absent mitral closing click

Disorder	Abnormal breath sounds	Abnormal heart sounds
Malfunctioning mitral prosthetic valve	▪ Inspiratory and expiratory crackles over the posterior lung bases associated with heart failure	▪ Holosystolic murmur ▪ New diastolic murmur or change in intensity or duration of existing one ▪ Diastolic rumble ▪ Absent mitral closing click
Mitral regurgitation	▪ Inspiratory and expiratory crackles over the posterior lung bases associated with heart failure	▪ Holosystolic murmur ▪ Decreased S_1 intensity ▪ Increased S_2 intensity ▪ Accented P_2 ▪ S_3 and S_4 ▪ Persistent A_2-P_2 splitting during expiration
Mitral stenosis		▪ With moderate stenosis, early and late diastolic murmur ▪ In severe stenosis, possibly holodiastolic murmur ▪ Loud M_1 ▪ Intensified S_1 except with a calcified valve, which produces a soft S_1 ▪ Split S_2 ▪ Opening snap except with a calcified valve ▪ S_3
Mitral valve prolapse		▪ Late systolic or holosystolic murmur ▪ Nonejection midsystolic click that's variable in intensity and timing ▪ Precordial honk
Myocardial infarction	▪ Inspiratory and expiratory crackles over the posterior lung bases associated with heart failure	▪ S_3 and S_4 ▪ S_1 and S_2 of faint and poor quality ▪ Paradoxical splitting S_2 with left ventricular dysfunction or left bundle branch block ▪ Physiologic splitting S_2 with right bundle branch block, ventricular septal defect, severe mitral regurgitation ▪ Harsh holosystolic murmur, crescendo–decrescendo with palpable thrill if ventricular septal rupture

(continued)

Disorder	Abnormal breath sounds	Abnormal heart sounds
Patent ductus arteriosus		▪ Continuous murmur reaching maximum intensity during late systole ▪ Murmur envelops S_2 ▪ Paradoxical S_2 split ▪ S_3 ▪ Diastolic flow rumble
Pericarditis		▪ Muffled heart sounds ▪ Pericardial friction rub, which has both a systolic (loudest) and diastolic component ▪ Scratchy, superficial quality
Pleural effusion	▪ Absent or diminished low-pitched breath sounds ▪ Occasionally loud bronchial breath sounds ▪ Normal breath sounds on contralateral side ▪ Bronchophony, egophony, and whispered pectoriloquy at upper border of pleural effusion	
Pneumonia	▪ High-pitched, tubular bronchial breath sounds heard over affected area during inspiration and expiration ▪ Bronchophony ▪ Egophony ▪ Whispered pectoriloquy ▪ Late inspiratory crackles not affected by coughing or position changes ▪ I:E ratio: 1:1	
Pneumothorax	▪ Absent or diminished low-pitched breath sounds ▪ Inaudible bronchophony, egophony, and whispered pectoriloquy ▪ Normal breath sounds heard on contralateral side	

Disorder	Abnormal breath sounds	Abnormal heart sounds
Pulmonary edema	• Inspiratory and expiratory crackles over the posterior lung bases; as pulmonary edema worsens, crackles are more profuse and heard during late inspiration • Wheezes	• S_3 or S_4
Pulmonic regurgitation		• Early diastolic murmur intensified during inspiration • Loud P_2
Pulmonic valve stenosis		• Midsystolic murmur • Systolic ejection click • P_2 absent or diminished and delayed • Normal or widened S_2 split • S_4
Supravalvular aortic stenosis		• Midsystolic murmur • Normal S_2 split • No aortic ejection sound
Tricuspid stenosis		• Mid- to late diastolic murmur, which increases during inspiration and fades during expiration • Normal S_2 or may be split during inspiration • Soft opening snap
Ventricular septal defect	• Crackles over posterior bases associated with heart failure	• Loud holosystolic murmur • Persistent A_2-P_2 splitting during expiration • S_3 followed by short low-frequency diastolic murmur • Pulmonic ejection sound • Loud P_2
Whooping cough	• Stridor	

Assessment flowcharts for common auscultation findings

These flowcharts will help you quickly recognize and provide interventions for seven common and, possibly, life-threatening findings. Each flowchart includes presenting signs and symptoms, diagnostic tests, treatment, and follow-up care.

Flowchart abbreviations

ABC	Airway, breathing, and circulation
ABG	Arterial blood gas
ACE	Angiotensin-converting enzyme
ARDS	Acute respiratory distress syndrome
AV	Atrioventricular
CBC	Complete blood count
CT	Computed tomography
CXR	Chest X-ray
DX	Diagnosis
ECG	Electrocardiogram
F/U	Follow-up
GERD	Gastroesophageal reflux disease
HEENT	Head, ears, eyes, nose, and throat
HPI	History of present illness
IABP	Intra-aortic balloon pump
I.V.	Intravenous
JVD	Jugular vein distention
MI	Myocardial infarction
MRI	Magnetic resonance imaging
PCI	Percutaneous coronary intervention
PE	Physical examination
PFT	Pulmonary function tests
SLE	Systemic lupus erythematosus
SOB	Shortness of breath
Sub-Q	Subcutaneous
Tc	Technetium
TX	Treatment
V̇/Q̇	Ventilation–perfusion

GALLOP, ATRIAL OR VENTRICULAR

An atrial gallop (S_4) is auscultated immediately before the first heart sound (S_1) and results from abnormal forceful atrial contraction caused by augmented ventricular filling or by decreased left ventricular compliance. A ventricular gallop (S_3) is auscultated immediately after the second heart sound (S_2) and results from rapid deceleration of blood entering a stiff, noncompliant ventricle or rapid acceleration of blood associated with increased flow into the ventricle. These two left ventricular sounds may be heard over the mitral area.

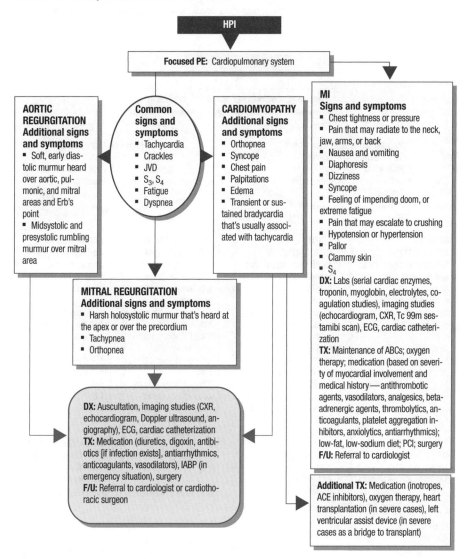

Additional differential diagnoses for atrial gallop: anemia ▪ angina ▪ aortic stenosis ▪ AV block ▪ hypertension ▪ pulmonary embolism

Additional differential diagnoses for ventricular gallop: heart failure ▪ thyrotoxicosis

MURMUR

Murmurs are auscultatory sounds heard within the heart chambers or major arteries. They're classified by their timing and duration in the cardiac cycle, auscultatory location, loudness, configuration, pitch, and quality.

Murmurs can reflect accelerated blood flow through a normal or an abnormal valve; forward blood flow through a narrowed or irregular valve or into a dilated vessel; blood backflow through an incompetent valve, septal defect, or patent ductus arteriosus; or decreased blood viscosity. Typically the result of organic heart disease, murmurs occasionally signal an emergency. Murmurs may also result from surgical implantation of a prosthetic valve.

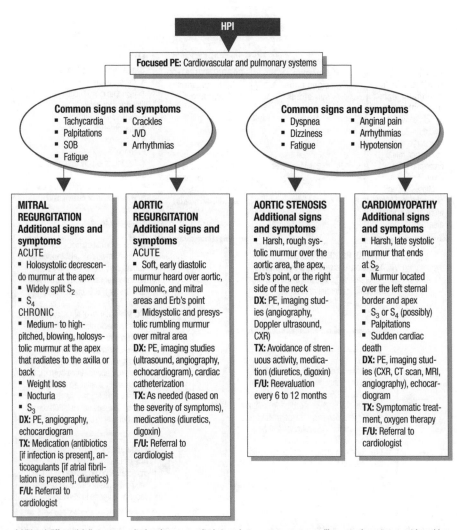

HPI

Focused PE: Cardiovascular and pulmonary systems

Common signs and symptoms
- Tachycardia
- Palpitations
- SOB
- Fatigue
- Crackles
- JVD
- Arrhythmias

Common signs and symptoms
- Dyspnea
- Dizziness
- Fatigue
- Anginal pain
- Arrhythmias
- Hypotension

MITRAL REGURGITATION
Additional signs and symptoms
ACUTE
- Holosystolic decrescendo murmur at the apex
- Widely split S_2
- S_4
CHRONIC
- Medium- to high-pitched, blowing, holosystolic murmur at the apex that radiates to the axilla or back
- Weight loss
- Nocturia
- S_3
DX: PE, angiography, echocardiogram
TX: Medication (antibiotics [if infection is present], anticoagulants [if atrial fibrillation is present], diuretics)
F/U: Referral to cardiologist

AORTIC REGURGITATION
Additional signs and symptoms
ACUTE
- Soft, early diastolic murmur heard over aortic, pulmonic, and mitral areas and Erb's point
- Midsystolic and presystolic rumbling murmur over mitral area
DX: PE, imaging studies (ultrasound, angiography, echocardiogram), cardiac catheterization
TX: As needed (based on the severity of symptoms), medications (diuretics, digoxin)
F/U: Referral to cardiologist

AORTIC STENOSIS
Additional signs and symptoms
- Harsh, rough systolic murmur over the aortic area, the apex, Erb's point, or the right side of the neck
DX: PE, imaging studies (angiography, Doppler ultrasound, CXR)
TX: Avoidance of strenuous activity, medication (diuretics, digoxin)
F/U: Reevaluation every 6 to 12 months

CARDIOMYOPATHY
Additional signs and symptoms
- Harsh, late systolic murmur that ends at S_2
- Murmur located over the left sternal border and apex
- S_3 or S_4 (possibly)
- Palpitations
- Sudden cardiac death
DX: PE, imaging studies (CXR, CT scan, MRI, angiography), echocardiogram
TX: Symptomatic treatment, oxygen therapy
F/U: Referral to cardiologist

Additional differential diagnoses: mitral prolapse ▪ mitral stenosis ▪ myxomas ▪ papillary muscle rupture ▪ tricuspid regurgitation ▪ tricuspid stenosis

Other causes: prosthetic valve replacement

CRACKLES

A common finding in certain cardiovascular and pulmonary diseases, crackles are characterized by short, explosive, or popping sounds usually heard during inspiration. They may be described as coarse (loud and low in pitch) or fine (less intense and high in pitch). Crackles are believed to result either when air bubbles through secretions in the airways or when the airways open suddenly and explosively.

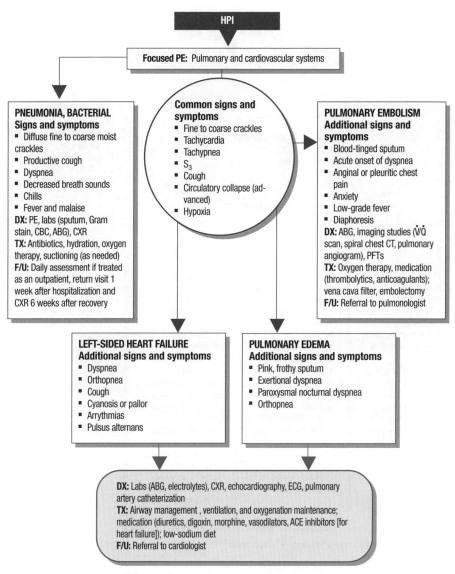

HPI

Focused PE: Pulmonary and cardiovascular systems

PNEUMONIA, BACTERIAL
Signs and symptoms
- Diffuse fine to coarse moist crackles
- Productive cough
- Dyspnea
- Decreased breath sounds
- Chills
- Fever and malaise

DX: PE, labs (sputum, Gram stain, CBC, ABG), CXR
TX: Antibiotics, hydration, oxygen therapy, suctioning (as needed)
F/U: Daily assessment if treated as an outpatient, return visit 1 week after hospitalization and CXR 6 weeks after recovery

Common signs and symptoms
- Fine to coarse crackles
- Tachycardia
- Tachypnea
- S_3
- Cough
- Circulatory collapse (advanced)
- Hypoxia

PULMONARY EMBOLISM
Additional signs and symptoms
- Blood-tinged sputum
- Acute onset of dyspnea
- Anginal or pleuritic chest pain
- Anxiety
- Low-grade fever
- Diaphoresis

DX: ABG, imaging studies ($\dot{V}/\dot{Q}$ scan, spiral chest CT, pulmonary angiogram), PFTs
TX: Oxygen therapy, medication (thrombolytics, anticoagulants); vena cava filter, embolectomy
F/U: Referral to pulmonologist

LEFT-SIDED HEART FAILURE
Additional signs and symptoms
- Dyspnea
- Orthopnea
- Cough
- Cyanosis or pallor
- Arrythmias
- Pulsus alternans

PULMONARY EDEMA
Additional signs and symptoms
- Pink, frothy sputum
- Exertional dyspnea
- Paroxysmal nocturnal dyspnea
- Orthopnea

DX: Labs (ABG, electrolytes), CXR, echocardiography, ECG, pulmonary artery catheterization
TX: Airway management, ventilation, and oxygenation maintenance; medication (diuretics, digoxin, morphine, vasodilators, ACE inhibitors [for heart failure]); low-sodium diet
F/U: Referral to cardiologist

Additional differential diagnoses: ARDS ▪ asthma (acute) ▪ bronchiectasis ▪ bronchitis (chronic) ▪ interstitial fibrosis of the lungs ▪ Legionnaire disease ▪ lung abscess ▪ pneumonia ▪ psittacosis ▪ pulmonary tuberculosis ▪ sarcoidosis ▪ silicosis ▪ tracheobronchitis

PLEURAL FRICTION RUB (PLEURAL CRACKLES)

Commonly resulting from a pulmonary disorder or trauma, pleural friction rub (or *pleural crackles*) is a coarse, grating sound that may be auscultated over one or both lungs during inspiration or expiration. Pleural friction rub indicates inflammation of the visceral and parietal pleural lining. The resultant fibrinous exudate causes the pleural surfaces to lose their ability to glide silently over each other during breathing. Patients with pleural friction rub typically have sharp inspiratory pain, causing them to splint the affected side in an attempt to reduce muscle and chest wall movement.

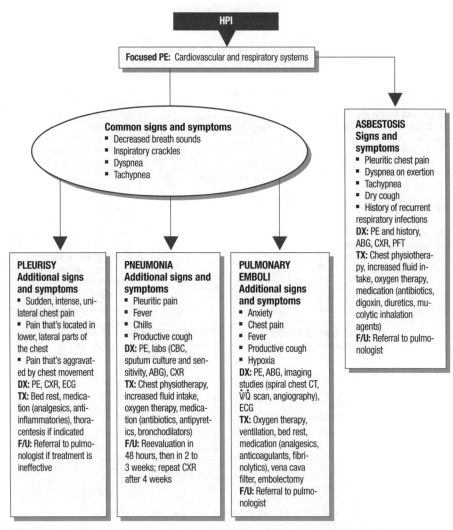

HPI

Focused PE: Cardiovascular and respiratory systems

Common signs and symptoms
- Decreased breath sounds
- Inspiratory crackles
- Dyspnea
- Tachypnea

ASBESTOSIS Signs and symptoms
- Pleuritic chest pain
- Dyspnea on exertion
- Tachypnea
- Dry cough
- History of recurrent respiratory infections

DX: PE and history, ABG, CXR, PFT
TX: Chest physiotherapy, increased fluid intake, oxygen therapy, medication (antibiotics, digoxin, diuretics, mucolytic inhalation agents)
F/U: Referral to pulmonologist

PLEURISY Additional signs and symptoms
- Sudden, intense, unilateral chest pain
- Pain that's located in lower, lateral parts of the chest
- Pain that's aggravated by chest movement

DX: PE, CXR, ECG
TX: Bed rest, medication (analgesics, antiinflammatories), thoracentesis if indicated
F/U: Referral to pulmonologist if treatment is ineffective

PNEUMONIA Additional signs and symptoms
- Pleuritic pain
- Fever
- Chills
- Productive cough

DX: PE, labs (CBC, sputum culture and sensitivity, ABG), CXR
TX: Chest physiotherapy, increased fluid intake, oxygen therapy, medication (antibiotics, antipyretics, bronchodilators)
F/U: Reevaluation in 48 hours, then in 2 to 3 weeks; repeat CXR after 4 weeks

PULMONARY EMBOLI Additional signs and symptoms
- Anxiety
- Chest pain
- Fever
- Productive cough
- Hypoxia

DX: PE, ABG, imaging studies (spiral chest CT, V̇/Q̇ scan, angiography), ECG
TX: Oxygen therapy, ventilation, bed rest, medication (analgesics, anticoagulants, fibrinolytics), vena cava filter, embolectomy
F/U: Referral to pulmonologist

Additional differential diagnoses: lung cancer ▪ rheumatoid arthritis ▪ SLE ▪ tuberculosis (pulmonary)

Other causes: radiation therapy ▪ thoracic surgery

LOW-PITCHED WHEEZES (RHONCHI)

Low-pitched wheezes, previously known as *sonorous rales* or *sonorous rhonchi*, are continuous and low-pitched, producing a snoring sound. The term *rhonchi* may still be used in the clinical setting to describe a rough, rumbling low-pitched sound heard mainly on expiration. Low-pitched wheezes are typically produced when fluid or secretions narrow the large airways, and often change in sound or disappear with coughing.

Additional differential diagnoses: asthma ▪ bronchiectasis ▪ pulmonary coccidioidomycosis

Other causes: bronchoscopy ▪ foreign body aspiration ▪ PFTs ▪ respiratory therapy

STRIDOR

A loud, musical respiratory sound, stridor results from an obstruction in the trachea or larynx and may be heard without a stethoscope. Usually heard during inspiration, this sign may also occur during expiration in severe upper-airway obstruction. Stridor may signal a life-threatening condition requiring prompt emergency interventions.

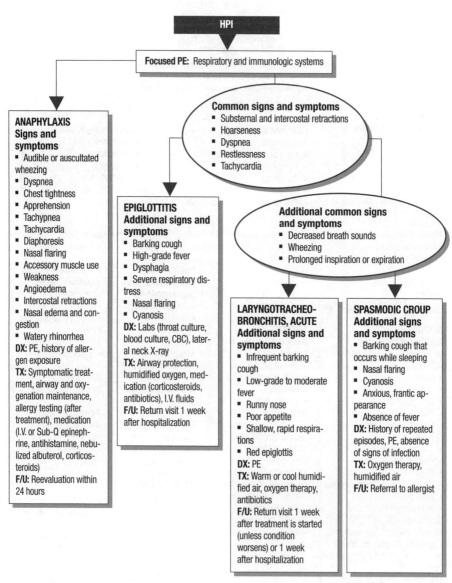

HPI

Focused PE: Respiratory and immunologic systems

ANAPHYLAXIS
Signs and symptoms
- Audible or auscultated wheezing
- Dyspnea
- Chest tightness
- Apprehension
- Tachypnea
- Tachycardia
- Diaphoresis
- Nasal flaring
- Accessory muscle use
- Weakness
- Angioedema
- Intercostal retractions
- Nasal edema and congestion
- Watery rhinorrhea
DX: PE, history of allergen exposure
TX: Symptomatic treatment, airway and oxygenation maintenance, allergy testing (after treatment), medication (I.V. or Sub-Q epinephrine, antihistamine, nebulized albuterol, corticosteroids)
F/U: Reevaluation within 24 hours

Common signs and symptoms
- Substernal and intercostal retractions
- Hoarseness
- Dyspnea
- Restlessness
- Tachycardia

EPIGLOTTITIS
Additional signs and symptoms
- Barking cough
- High-grade fever
- Dysphagia
- Severe respiratory distress
- Nasal flaring
- Cyanosis
DX: Labs (throat culture, blood culture, CBC), lateral neck X-ray
TX: Airway protection, humidified oxygen, medication (corticosteroids, antibiotics), I.V. fluids
F/U: Return visit 1 week after hospitalization

Additional common signs and symptoms
- Decreased breath sounds
- Wheezing
- Prolonged inspiration or expiration

LARYNGOTRACHEO-BRONCHITIS, ACUTE
Additional signs and symptoms
- Infrequent barking cough
- Low-grade to moderate fever
- Runny nose
- Poor appetite
- Shallow, rapid respirations
- Red epiglottis
DX: PE
TX: Warm or cool humidified air, oxygen therapy, antibiotics
F/U: Return visit 1 week after treatment is started (unless condition worsens) or 1 week after hospitalization

SPASMODIC CROUP
Additional signs and symptoms
- Barking cough that occurs while sleeping
- Nasal flaring
- Cyanosis
- Anxious, frantic appearance
- Absence of fever
DX: History of repeated episodes, PE, absence of signs of infection
TX: Oxygen therapy, humidified air
F/U: Referral to allergist

Additional differential diagnoses: airway trauma ▪ hypocalcemia ▪ inhalation injury ▪ laryngeal tumor ▪ mediastinal tumor ▪ retrosternal thyroid ▪ thoracic aortic aneurysm

Other causes: bronchoscopy ▪ foreign body aspiration ▪ laryngoscopy ▪ neck surgery ▪ prolonged intubation

WHEEZING

Wheezes are high-pitched, continuous musical sounds that result when air passes rapidly through a narrowed bronchus that oscillates between being barely open to being completely closed. The causes of airway narrowing include bronchospasm; obstructive lung disease; mucosal thickening or edema; partial obstruction from a tumor, foreign body, or secretions; use of a β-adrenergic blocker; and extrinsic pressure, as in tension pneumothorax or goiter. Wheezing may signal a medical emergency requiring immediate medical intervention.

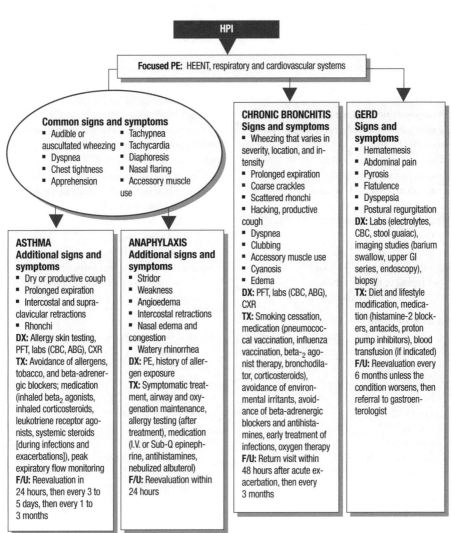

Additional differential diagnoses: aspiration of a foreign body ▪ aspiration pneumonitis ▪ bronchial adenoma ▪ bronchiectasis ▪ bronchogenic carcinoma ▪ chemical pneumonitis (acute) ▪ emphysema ▪ inhalation injury ▪ pneumothorax (tension) ▪ pulmonary coccidioidomycosis ▪ pulmonary edema ▪ pulmonary embolus ▪ pulmonary tuberculosis ▪ thyroid goiter ▪ tracheobronchitis ▪ Wegener granulomatosis

English–Spanish phrases used in cardiac and respiratory assessment

HEALTH PROBLEMS

Chest pain

General

Have you ever had chest pain or discomfort?

¿Ha tenido Ud. alguna vez dolor de pecho o molestias?

Description

–How is the pain?
  Constant?
  Intermittent?
Do any activities produce the pain?
Does it hurt when you breathe normally or when you breathe deeply?
What does the pain feel like?
  –Crushing or squeezing?
  –Someone or something heavy pressing on your chest?
  –Pressure or tightness?
  –Dull ache?
  –Burning sensation?
  –Sharp or stabbing like a knife?
  – Ripping or tearing sensation?
  – Heartburn-type pain?

–¿Cómo lo describiría?
  ¿Constante?
  ¿Intermitente?
¿Qué actividad o actividades le producen el dolor?
¿Le duele a Ud. cuando respira normalmente o cuando respira profundamente?
¿Qué clase de dolor siente?
  –¿Siente que lo aplasta u oprime?
  –¿Tiene la sensación de que alguien o algo pesado le oprime el pecho?
  –¿Siente presión o tensión?
  –¿Es un dolor sordo?
  –¿Es un dolor urente?
  –¿Es agudo o punzante como un cuchillo?
  –¿Siente que es un dolor desgarrante?
  –¿Siente sensación de ardor en el pecho?

Other symptoms

Do you have any other symptoms with the pain?
  –Anxiety?
  –Dizziness?
  –Fainting?
  –Feeling of doom?
  –Jaw pain?
  –Nausea?
  –Restlessness?
  –Shortness of breath?
  –Sweating?
  –Vomiting?
  –Weakness?

¿Tiene otros síntomas además del dolor?
  –¿Ansiedad?
  –¿Mareos?
  –¿Desmayos?
  –¿Depresión?
  –¿Dolor mandibular?
  –¿Náuseas?
  –¿Inquietud?
  –¿Respiración dificultosa?
  –¿Sudor?
  –¿Vómitos?
  –¿Debilidad?

Aggravating factors

Does anything make the pain worse?
  –Standing?
  –Walking?
  –Climbing stairs?

¿Hay algo que empeore el dolor?
  –¿Pararse?
  –¿Caminar?
  –¿Subir escaleras?

Alleviating factors

Does anything make the pain better?	¿Hay algo que alivie el dolor?
–Lying down?	–¿Acostarse?
–Resting?	–¿Descansar?
–Taking medication?	–¿Tomar medicamentos?

Location

Where in your chest do you feel the pain?	¿En qué parte del pecho siente Ud. el dolor?
Can you point to where you feel the pain?	¿Puede Ud. señalar con el dedo dónde siente el dolor?
–Does it radiate to any other area?	–¿Se irradia este dolor a otra parte del cuerpo?

Duration

How long have you been having this chest pain?	¿Cuánto tiempo hace que tiene Ud. este dolor de pecho?
–Did it start recently?	–¿Comenzó hace poco?
–Over the last few hours, days, or weeks?	–¿En las últimas horas, días o semanas?
How long does an attack last?	¿Cuánto tiempo dura un ataque?
–Seconds?	–¿Segundos?
–Minutes?	–¿Minutos?
–Hours?	–¿Horas?
–Days?	–¿Días?

Arrhythmias

Does your heart ever feel like it's:	¿Siente Ud. alguna vez que el corazón:
–pounding?	–le late violentamente?
–racing?	–le late aceleradamente?
–skipping beats?	–omite latidos?
When does this feeling occur?	¿Cuándo tiene esta sensación?
–While resting?	–¿Mientras descansa?
–During an activity?	–¿Mientras lleva a cabo alguna actividad?
–After an activity?	–¿Después de desempeñar una actividad?
–After exercising?	–¿Después de hacer ejercicio?
–After walking up steps?	–¿Después de subir la escalera?
–After eating?	–¿Después de comer?

Cough

General

Do you have a cough?	¿Tiene Ud. tos?

Description

What does it sound like?	¿De qué tipo es?
Hacking?	¿Tos seca?
Barking?	¿Tos perruna?
Congested?	¿Congestionada?

Timing

Does it usually occur at a certain time of day?	Por lo general, ¿aparece a cierta hora del día?
–When?	–¿Cuándo?

Sputum production

Do you cough up sputum?	¿Expectora Ud.?
–How much do you cough up each day?	¿Cuánto expectora Ud. al día?
–What color is it?	–¿De qué color es?
Red?	¿Rojo?
Pink?	¿Rosado?
With streaks of blood?	¿Sanguinolento?
Yellow?	¿Amarillo?
Green?	¿Verde?
White?	¿Blanco?
Clear?	¿Transparente o claro?
–How does it smell?	–¿Qué olor tiene?
–Is it thick?	–¿Es el esputo denso?
–Is it thin?	–¿Es el esputo claro?
–What time of day do you cough up the most sputum?	–¿A qué hora del día expectora Ud. más?
Morning?	¿Por la mañana?
Night?	¿Por la noche?
After meals?	¿Después de las comidas?

Breathing difficulties

General

Do you have shortness of breath?	¿Tiene Ud. dificultad para respirar?

Description

When did it occur?	¿Cuándo le ocurrió?
Is it constant?	¿Es constante?
Is it intermittent?	¿Es intermitente?
What makes it better?	¿Qué mejora la respiracion?
What makes it worse?	¿Qué la empeora?
Does position, medication, or relaxation relieve it?	¿Le alivia a Ud. el descanso, algún medicamento, o el cambio de postura?
Is shortness of breath related to any activity?	¿Está relacionada la dificultad respiratoria con alguna actividad?
–Which activity?	–¿Con qué actividad?
Is shortness of breath accompanied by coughing?	¿Se acompaña la dificultad respiratoria de tos?
Do your lips or nail beds ever turn blue?	¿Alguna vez se le ponen azulados los labios o los lechos ungueales?
Does body position affect your breathing?	¿Afecta a la respiración la postura del cuerpo?
–How?	–¿Cómo?
Does time of day affect your breathing?	¿Le afecta la hora del día a la respiración?
–What time of day?	–¿A qué hora del día se siente peor?
How many stairs can you climb before you feel short of breath?	¿Cuántos escalones puede Ud. subir antes de sentir que le falta al aliento?
How many blocks can you walk before you feel short of breath?	¿Cuántas travesías puede recorrer antes de sentir que le falta el aliento?

Fatigue
General

Do you tire more easily than you used to?	¿Se cansa Ud. con más facilidad que antes?
What type of activity causes you to feel fatigued?	¿Qué tipo de actividad le hace sentirse fatigado/a?
–How long can you perform this activity before you feel fatigued?	–¿Durante cuánto tiempo puede Ud. realizar esa actividad antes de sentirse fatigado?
–Does rest relieve the fatigue?	–¿El reposo le mitiga la fatiga?

Swelling
General

Do your shoes or rings feel tight?	¿Le aprietan los zapatos o los anillos?
Do your ankles or feet feel swollen?	¿Siente Ud. que se le hinchan los tobillos o los pies?
How long have you felt this way?	¿Cuánto tiempo hace que se siente así?
Have you gained or lost weight recently?	¿Aumentó o perdió peso recientemente?

Respiratory treatments
Medications

Do you ever use over-the-counter nasal sprays or inhalers?	¿Usa Ud. alguna vez atomizadores nasales o inhaladores?
–What kind do you use?	–¿Qué clase usa Ud.?
–How frequently do you use them?	–¿Con qué frecuencia los usa?
Do you take any over-the-counter or prescription drugs for your respiratory difficulties?	¿Toma Ud. medicamentos con o sin receta médica para sus dificultades respiratorias?
–Which drugs?	–¿Qué medicamentos?
–Any steroids?	–¿Esteroides?
–How often do you take them?	–¿Con qué frecuencia los toma Ud.?
–When did you last take these drugs?	–¿Cuándo fue la última vez que tomó estos medicamentos?
Do you use a nebulizer or other breathing treatment?	¿Usa Ud. un nebulizador u otro tratamiento para respirar?
–What condition does it treat?	–¿Para qué enfermedad lleva Ud. a cabo el tratamiento?
–What dose do you use?	–¿Qué dosis se le dio?
–How often do you have a treatment?	–¿Con qué frecuencia sigue Ud. un tratamiento?

Oxygen

Do you use oxygen at home?	¿Usa Ud. oxígeno en casa?
–Do you use a cannula or a mask?	–¿Usa Ud. una cánula o máscara?
–How often do you use it?	–¿Con qué frecuencia la usa?
Continuously?	¿Continuamente?
Intermittently?	¿Intermitentemente?

MEDICAL HISTORY

Cardiovascular history
General

Were you born with a heart problem?	¿Nació Ud. con algún problema cardiaco?
–When was it treated?	–¿Cuándo recibió tratamiento?
–How was it treated?	–¿Cómo se le trató?

Rheumatic fever

Have you had rheumatic fever?	¿Ha tenido Ud. fiebre reumática?
When?	–¿Cuándo?
Have any heart problems resulted from the rheumatic fever?	¿Ha sufrido algún problema cardiaco debido a la fiebre reumática?

Heart murmur

Have you ever been told you had a heart murmur?	¿Le han dicho alguna vez que tenía un soplo cardiaco?
–Who told you about it?	–¿Quién se lo dijo?
–When did you find out about it?	–¿Cuándo se enteró Ud. de ello?

Other conditions

Do you have any of the following conditions?	¿Padece Ud. alguna de las siguientes enfermedades?
–High blood pressure?	–¿Presión sanguínea alta?
–High cholesterol?	–¿Colesterol alto?
–Diabetes mellitus?	–¿Diabetes mellitus?
–Heart failure?	–¿Insuficiencia cardiaca?
When was the disorder first diagnosed?	¿Cuándo se le diagnosticó por primera vez este trastorno?
How do you manage it?	¿Cómo lo controla?
How has it affected your lifestyle?	¿Cómo ha influido en su modo de vida?

Procedures

Have you ever had _____?	¿Se ha sometido alguna vez a _____?
–a cardiac catheterization	–una cateterización cardiaca
–a stent placed	–la colocación de una endoprotésis (stent)
–an angioplasty	–una angioplastia
–any type of heart surgery	–algún tipo de cirugía cardiaca
–a pacemaker inserted	–la colocación de un marcapasos
–a defibrillator inserted	–la colocación de un desfibrilador

Respiratory history
General

Have you had any lung problems?	¿Ha tenido Ud. algún problema pulmonar?
–Asthma?	–¿Asma?
–Tuberculosis?	–¿Tuberculosis?
–Pneumonia?	–¿Pulmonía?
–Influenza?	–¿Gripe?
–Sinus problems?	–¿Sinusitis?

–Emphysema?

–Allergies?

–Other?

How long did the problem last?

How was the problem treated?

–¿Enfisema?

–¿Alergias?

–¿Otros?

¿Cuánto tiempo le duró el problema?

¿Qué tratamiento recibió?

Exposure history

Have you been exposed to anyone with a respiratory disease?

–What type of disease?

–When were you exposed?

Are there any respiratory irritants in your home, such as fresh paint, cleaning sprays, or heavy cigarette smoke?

¿Ha estado Ud. expuesto/a a alguna persona que tenga una enfermedad respiratoria?

–¿Qué clase de enfermedad?

–¿Cuándo estuvo Ud. expuesto/a?

¿Hay en su casa sustancias irritantes que le afecten a la respiración, tales como superficies recién pintadas, productos de limpieza en aerosol o humo de cigarrillos?

Diagnostic tests

Have you had a diagnostic study of the lungs?

–What type?

–Why did you have it?

When was your last chest X-ray?

When was your last tuberculosis test?

–What was the result?

¿Le han hecho algún examen de los pulmones?

–¿De qué tipo?

–¿Por qué motivo se lo hicieron?

¿Cuándo fue la última vez que le hicieron una radiografía de tórax?

¿Cuándo fue la última vez que le hicieron una prueba para la tuberculosis?

–¿Cuál fue el resultado?

Procedures

Have you had chest surgery?

Have you had surgery on your___?

–lungs

–sinuses

–mouth, nose, or throat

¿Lo han operado del pecho?

¿Le han operado_____?

–de los pulmones

–de los senos nasales

–de la boca, la nariz o la garganta

Allergies

Do you have allergies that flare up in different seasons?

–What causes them?

–Do they cause any of these symptoms:

runny nose?

itching eyes?

congestion?

other symptoms?

–What do you do to relieve these symptoms?

In the last 2 months, have you had:

–fever?

–chills?

–fatigue?

–night sweats?

¿Tiene Ud. alergias que se agravan en las distintas estaciones del año?

–¿Qué es lo que las causa?

–¿Le producen alguno de los siguientes síntomas:

¿le gotea la nariz?

¿le pican los ojos?

¿tiene congestión?

¿otros síntomas?

–¿Qué hace Ud. para aliviar estos síntomas?

¿En los últimos dos meses ha tenido:

–¿fiebre?

–¿escalofríos?

–¿fatiga?

–¿sudores nocturnos?

FAMILY HISTORY

Has anyone in your family been treated for heart disease?	¿Algún miembro de su familia ha recibido tratamiento para alguna enfermedad cardiaca?
Has anyone in your family died suddenly of an unknown cause?	¿Algún miembro de su familia ha fallecido repentinamente por causa desconocida?
Has any member of your family had:	¿Algún miembro de su familia padeció alguna de las siguientes enfermedades:

 –emphysema?   –¿enfisema?
 –asthma?   –¿asma?
 –respiratory allergies?   –¿alergias respiratorias?
 –tuberculosis?   –¿tuberculosis?
 –sarcoidosis?   –¿sarcoidosis?

Did you have contact with the family member who had tuberculosis?	¿Estuvo Ud. en contacto con el miembro de la familia que tuvo tuberculosis?

 –When?   –¿Cuándo?
 –Do they live with you?   –¿Vive con Ud.?

LIFESTYLE

Tobacco

Do you smoke or chew tobacco?	¿Fuma o masca Ud. tabaco?
–What do you smoke?	–¿Qué fuma?
Cigarettes?	¿Cigarrillos?
Cigars?	¿Cigarros (puros)?
Pipes?	¿En pipa?
–How long have you smoked or chewed tobacco?	–¿Cuánto tiempo hace que fuma o masca tabaco?
–How many cigarettes, cigars, or pipes of tobacco do you smoke per day?	–¿Cuántos cigarrillos, cigarros (puros) o pipas de tabaco fuma Ud. al día?

Alcohol

Do you drink alcoholic beverages?	¿Toma Ud. bebidas alcohólicas?
–What type?	–¿De qué clase?
Beer?	¿Cerveza?
Wine?	¿Vino?
Hard liquor?	¿Licores o aguardientes?
How often do you drink?	¿Con qué frecuencia bebe Ud.?
How many drinks per day?	¿Qué cantidad bebe al día?

Sleep patterns

Do you awaken during the night to urinate?	¿Se despierta Ud. durante la noche para orinar?
Do you ever have shortness of breath or coughing spells during the night?	¿Alguna vez tiene dificultad para respirar o sufre accesos de tos por la noche?
Do you become short of breath when you lie flat?	¿Tiene Ud. dificultad para respirar cuando se acuesta sobre la espalda?
How many pillows do you use at night?	¿Cuántas almohadas usa Ud. por la noche?

Have your sleep patterns changed because of breathing problems?

¿Han cambiado sus hábitos de sueño a causa de sus problemas respiratorios?

Exercise

Do you exercise routinely?
  –How often do you exercise?
  –How intensely do you exercise?
  –How long do you spend exercising?

¿Hace Ud. ejercicio rutinariamente?
  –¿Con qué frecuencia hace ejercicio?
  –¿Con qué intensidad hace el ejercicio?
  –¿Durante cuánto tiempo hace Ud. ejercicio?

Stress

How often do you experience stress?
  –Rarely?
  –Once in a while?
  –Very often?
Are you ever overwhelmed by stress?

¿Con qué frecuencia siente Ud. estrés?
  –¿Raramente?
  –¿De vez en cuando?
  –¿Con frecuencia?
¿Se siente Ud. alguna vez abrumado/a por el estrés?

Employment

Are you currently employed?
What's your occupation?
What were your previous occupations?
Are you exposed to any known respiratory irritants at work?
  –Do you use safety measures during exposure?

¿Tiene Ud. empleo actualmente?
¿Cuál es su profesión o trabajo?
¿Qué otros empleos ha tenido anteriormente?
¿Sabe Ud. si en su trabajo está expuesto a sustancias irritantes que afecten a su respiración?
  –¿Usa Ud. medidas de seguridad mientras está expuesto/a?

Posttest answers

HEART SOUNDS

1 The heart and auscultation

1. The heart's primary function is to pump deoxygenated blood to the lungs, where carbon dioxide–oxygen (CO_2–O_2) exchange takes place, and to pump oxygenated blood throughout the body.

2. Anatomically, the heart is divided into two functional sides: the right side and the left side, which are separated by the septum. Each side is further divided into chambers. The right atrium and right ventricle are the right-sided chambers; the left atrium and left ventricle, the left-sided chambers.

3. The right atrioventricular, or tricuspid, valve separates the right atrium and right ventricle, and the left atrioventricular, or mitral, valve separates the left atrium and left ventricle. The semilunar pulmonic valve separates the right ventricle and pulmonary artery, and the semilunar aortic valve separates the left ventricle and aorta.

4. During systole, heart muscle contraction raises the intracardiac pressures enough to systematically open the valves and pump a certain volume of blood. During diastole, the heart muscle relaxes, allowing the chambers to fill with blood again. This entire sequence is called the cardiac cycle.

5. Cardiac output, the amount of blood pumped into the aorta each minute, depends largely on stroke volume. Stroke volume is the amount of blood pumped during each ventricular contraction.

6. Electrical impulses are primarily responsible for the heart's rhythmic pumping action. These impulses are discharged automatically from specialized cardiac cells that stimulate the heart muscle to contract. The specialized cardiac cells and fibers within the conduction system work together to produce a contraction. The impulses fired from the sinoatrial (SA) node, located just below the entrance of the superior vena cava in the right atrium, normally initiate the cardiac cycle, and they usually travel along specific pathways. For example, when the electrical impulse leaves the SA node, it travels along the atrial conduction pathways located in the atrial walls, initiating atrial systole (or atrial contraction). The impulse rapidly reaches the atrioventricular (AV) node, located near the AV junction. From the AV node, the impulse travels to the bundle of His, located in the interventricular septum. Here the bundle of His divides into the right and left bundle branches. These branches further divide into the tiny Purkinje fibers located throughout the ventricular walls. As the impulse travels through the bundle branches and Purkinje fibers, it initiates ventricular systole (or ventricular contraction).

7. The sequential and synchronized contraction (systole) and relaxation (diastole) of the atria and ventricles, along with the opening and closing of competent, properly functioning valves, ensure a unidirectional flow of blood through the heart and allow the heart to effectively move blood to all areas of the body quickly and repeatedly.

8. The aortic area is located at the second right intercostal space close to the sternal border. Abbreviated as 2RSB, this area is where the sounds of the aortic valve and aorta are heard best.

The pulmonic area is located at the second left intercostal space close to the sternal border. Abbreviated as 2LSB, this area is where the sounds of the pulmonic valve and pulmonary artery are heard best.

The tricuspid area is located at the fifth left intercostal space close to the sternal border. This area, abbreviated as 5LSB, is where the sounds of the tricuspid valve and right ventricle are heard best.

The mitral area is located at or near the fifth intercostal space just medial to the left midclavicular line. This area, directly over the left ventricle, is sometimes referred to as the apical area, or apex. The mitral area, abbreviated as 5LMCL, is where the sounds of the mitral valve and left ventricle are heard best.

Erb point differs from the other four areas in that it isn't named after a heart valve, but it's a good location to hear the sounds of aortic and pulmonic origin. Abbreviated as 3LSB, this area is located at the third left intercostal space close to the sternal border.

9. To use the diaphragm, firmly grasp the metal area between the bell and the diaphragm with your finger and thumb, and press down firmly on the chest wall. Or place your fingertips on the bell's rim, and press down firmly against the chest wall. Apply enough pressure so that an indentation remains on the skin after you remove the stethoscope.

The bell, however, should touch the chest wall only lightly. If you exert too much pressure when listening with the bell, the stretched skin beneath it will act as a diaphragm, filtering out low-pitched sounds. To hold the bell correctly, grasp the diaphragm's outer edges with the index finger and thumb, and gently rest the bell on the chest wall. Look at the skin around the edges of the bell to see if too much pressure is being applied. If any signs of indentation appear on the skin, relax the downward pressure.

10. Listen first with the diaphragm over the aortic area. Try to recognize the characteristic *lub-dub* sound of each cardiac cycle. After listening through several cycles, inch the diaphragm toward the pulmonic area. Try to move the diaphragm without losing track of the *lub-dub.* Then listen over the pulmonic area, Erb point, and the tricuspid area. Continue in this manner until you reach the mitral area.

2 Heart sound dynamics

1. S_1, the first heart sound, is heard at the beginning of systole. It's associated with the closure of the mitral and tricuspid valves and the increasing pressures within the ventricles that cause the moving valve leaflets and cord structures to decelerate. S_1 is generated by the closing atrioventricular valves and the vibrations associated with tensing of the chordae tendineae and ventricular walls.

2. At the end of ventricular systole, ventricular pressures fall rapidly, causing a slight backflow of blood from the aorta and pulmonary artery. The decrease in ventricular pressures to a level below that of aortic and pulmonic systolic pressures and the temporary backflow of blood and recoil events are associated with the closure of the aortic and pulmonic valves. The vibrations associated with these events produce the second heart sound, S_2, which marks the end of ventricular systole.

3. A sound's location is the anatomic area on the patient's chest wall where the sound is heard best. Bony structures and landmarks, such as the sternum and left midclavicular line, are used to describe the precise location.

4. Intensity refers to the sound's loudness during auscultation. Usually, a sound's intensity is determined subjectively, on the basis of experience. However, when abnormalities are present, intensity can be determined electronically by recording a phonocardiogram and measuring the amplitude of the sound's vibrations.

5. Sound duration refers to the length of time the sound is heard; it can be described as either short or long. A sound's duration affects whether you hear it as a click, a thud, or a snap.

6. A sound's pitch is determined by the frequency of its vibrations. High-frequency sounds, like the notes of a piccolo, are best

heard with the diaphragm of the stethoscope; low-frequency sounds, like the notes of a tuba, are best heard with the bell of the stethoscope.

7. Sound quality is determined by the combination of its frequencies. It may be described as sharp, dull, booming, or snapping.

8. A sound's timing refers to when it is heard during the cardiac cycle (during systole or diastole).

9. The electrocardiogram (ECG) correlates with the heart's electrical activity in the following manner: The sinoatrial node fires, and the impulse spreads through the atria. The P wave, part of the ECG waveform, represents atrial depolarization. Atrial contraction is stimulated by—and closely follows—atrial depolarization. The QRS complex represents electrical depolarization of the ventricles. Atrial repolarization isn't seen in the ECG because it's hidden in the P-R segment and the QRS complex. The T wave represents ventricular repolarization. The impulse travels through the atrioventricular node, the bundle of His, the bundle branches, and the Purkinje fibers before the ventricles contract. The time between atrial depolarization and ventricular depolarization is recorded in the ECG as the P-R interval: it begins at the onset of the P wave and lasts until the onset of the QRS complex. The time interval of the P-R interval correlates with the time interval between atrial contraction and ventricular contraction.

10. The first (S_1) and second (S_2) heart sounds directly correlate with a patient's ECG. S_1 normally occurs just after the QRS complex; S_2 occurs at the end of the T wave.

3 The first heart sound

1. The cardiac vibrations associated with the closure of the mitral and tricuspid valves produce the first heart sound, S_1.

2. Normally, only two components of the first heart sound are audible. The first component, referred to as M_1, is associated with the closure of the mitral valve; the second component, T_1, is associated with the closure of the tricuspid valve. Both valves close at the beginning of ventricular systole, but the mitral valve usually closes slightly ahead of the tricuspid valve.

3. M_1 and T_1 are usually perceived as a single sound called S_1, which is heard best near the heart's apex over the mitral area using the diaphragm of the stethoscope. A single sound is heard because left heart sounds are normally more intense at this site. S_1 occurs shortly after the beginning of the QRS complex in the ECG waveform. As you inch the stethoscope from the mitral area toward the tricuspid area, without losing track of S_1, the M_1 and T_1 components of S_1 become evident. Expiration may make them easier to hear. T_1 trails M_1 slightly and is softer; it's heard best near the left sternal border. The timing of M_1 and T_1 with the QRS complex remains the same. In many patients, only one first heart sound is heard because M_1 and T_1 are separated by ≤20 milliseconds, which the human ear perceives as one sound.

4. S_1 is usually heard best near the heart's apex over the mitral area. Its intensity directly relates to the force of ventricular contraction and the ECG P-R interval. The shorter the P-R interval, the more widely open are the mitral and tricuspid leaflets at the onset of ventricular contraction. Thus, the distance they must be moved is greater, resulting in more intense vibrations when they close and a louder S_1. S_1 is short in duration. You can hear its high pitch best using the diaphragm of the stethoscope. The quality of S_1 is somewhat dull. The S_1 timing coincides with the beginning of ventricular systole and just precedes a palpable carotid pulse.

5. S_1 can be enhanced by sympathetic stimulation, such as that provided by a brief period of exercise.

6. The normal M_1-T_1 split heard over the tricuspid area widens when electrical activation and contraction of the right ventricle

are delayed. Such a delay causes delayed tricuspid valve closure.

7. The conditions associated with an abnormal S_1 split are complete right bundle branch block, left ventricular ectopic beats, epicardial pacing of the left ventricle, tricuspid stenosis, atrial septal defect, Ebstein anomaly, and left ventricular tachycardia.

4 The second heart sound

1. The cardiac vibrations associated with the closure of the aortic and pulmonic valves produce the second heart sound, S_2.

2. S_2, like S_1, has two basic components: the aortic (A_2) component and the pulmonic (P_2) component. Both valves close at the end of ventricular systole. Normally, the aortic valve closes slightly ahead of the pulmonic valve.

3. To hear both components of S_2, listen carefully over the pulmonic area using the diaphragm of the stethoscope. Listen for S_2 just after the T wave in the patient's ECG.

4. S_2 is usually heard best near the heart's base over the pulmonic area or over Erb point. Its intensity directly relates to the amount of closing pressure in the aorta and pulmonary artery. S_2 is slightly shorter in duration than S_1. You can hear its high pitch best using the diaphragm of the stethoscope. The quality of S_2 is somewhat booming; its timing coincides with the end of ventricular systole.

5. The splitting of S_2 into the A_2 and P_2 components is heard best during inspiration over Erb point. Remember, inspiration causes an increase in the venous return to the right side of the heart. This increased venous return prolongs the right ventricular ejection time. Also, inspiration reduces pressure in the pulmonary artery. Both result in a delayed P_2, or closure of the pulmonic valve. A decrease in blood flow to the left side of the heart occurs simultaneously, resulting in a shorter left ventricular ejection time. Therefore, A_2 is heard earlier than P_2. This means that a normal S_2 split is heard during inspiration, and the A_2 and P_2 components fuse during expiration.

6. Abnormal splitting is related to valvular dysfunction, to alterations in blood flow to or from the ventricles, or to both. These changes may cause the normal S_2 split to be absent during both phases of the respiratory cycle. Thus, only a single S_2 is heard over Erb point. In another case, the split sounds may persist through inspiration and expiration with little or no respiratory variation. The split sounds may also be heard paradoxically on expiration. The A_2-P_2 intervals vary, as does the intensity of A_2 and P_2 during the respiratory cycle. Changes in S_2 splits are usually most noticeable at the beginning of inspiration and expiration.

7. The P_2 component may not be heard during auscultation over Erb point in the patient with severe pulmonic stenosis. Consequently, S_2 remains a single sound during both inspiration and expiration. A normal S_2 split may also be absent if the A_2 sound masks the P_2 sound or vice versa—for example, when one sound is significantly louder than the other, making splitting inaudible. This phenomenon occurs in patients with pulmonary hypertension. On the other hand, systemic hypertension causes A_2 to be delayed and to fuse with P_2 during inspiration.

8. A persistent S_2 split occurs when A_2 and P_2 don't fuse into one sound during expiration, even though some respiratory variation in the intensity of A_2 and P_2 is heard. This persistent A_2-P_2 splitting during expiration usually results from early aortic valve closure or delayed pulmonic valve closure. Early aortic valve closure is associated with shortened left ventricular systole, which occurs in patients with mitral regurgitation, ventricular septal defects, or cardiac tamponade. Delayed pulmonic valve closure occurs when right ventricular systole is prolonged in patients with chronic pulmonary hypertension. In these

patients, the A_2-P_2 split persists through inspiration and expiration, but the interval between the A_2 and P_2 components is more narrow than it is in a persistent S_2 split.

Another cause of persistent A_2-P_2 splitting throughout expiration is delayed electrical activation of the right ventricle, which delays P_2. This phenomenon is commonly found in patients with right bundle branch block, left ventricular epicardial pacing, or left ventricular ectopic beats.

9. A prolonged right ventricular ejection time produces expiratory A_2-P_2 splits that are widened and that persist even when the patient is seated. This occurs in patients with atrial septal defects, acute pulmonary hypertension secondary to massive pulmonary emboli, or pulmonic stenosis. The P_2 component may not be audible at all in patients with severe pulmonic stenosis. A wide, fixed S_2 split is sometimes associated with the pulmonary vascular bed's increased capacitance (ability to receive blood volume and the decreased resistance that accompanies it). This phenomenon occurs in patients with idiopathic dilation of the pulmonary artery or with atrial septal defects. This split doesn't change with respiration.

10. In a paradoxical, or reversed, S_2 split, P_2 precedes A_2, and the split sounds are heard during expiration instead of inspiration. This phenomenon is almost always caused by delayed aortic valve closure. If A_2 is delayed during expiration, it may follow P_2, causing an S_2 split; if A_2 is delayed during inspiration, A_2 and P_2 fuse because inspiration normally delays P_2. Therefore, S_2 is heard as a single sound during inspiration instead of a normally split sound.

Delayed A_2 is commonly seen in patients with delayed activation of the left ventricle caused by left bundle branch block. It's also associated with right ventricular ectopic beats or right ventricular endocardial pacing. Prolonged left ventricular systole can also cause a delay in

A_2. The same paradoxical P_2-A_2 split may be heard in patients with left-sided heart failure or ischemic heart disease.

Left ventricular pressure overload, which occurs in patients with systemic hypertension or hypertrophic cardiomyopathy, may also cause paradoxical S_2 split. Likewise, aortic stenosis may lead to paradoxical splitting of A_2 and P_2; however, if the stenosis is severe, the A_2 component may not be audible. With left ventricular volume overload, which is commonly associated with aortic regurgitation or patent ductus arteriosus, A_2 may be delayed, and a paradoxical S_2 split may be heard.

5 The third and fourth heart sounds

1. Early in diastole, after isovolumic relaxation, the mitral and tricuspid valves open and the ventricles fill and expand. In children and young adults, the left ventricle is normally compliant, permitting rapid filling. The left ventricle responds to this rapid filling with an abrupt change in wall motion that causes a sudden decrease in blood flow. These events generate vibrations that are responsible for the physiologic S_3.

2. S_3 is usually heard best over the mitral area using the bell of the stethoscope, and it can typically be palpated over the same area. It's heard best during expiration, when blood flow into the left ventricle is increased.

3. S_3 is usually heard best near the heart's apex over the mitral area. In some patients, it's faint in intensity and difficult to hear; in others, it's loud and easy to hear. S_3 has a short duration, and it may occur only intermittently during every third or fourth heartbeat. It has a low pitch that's heard best using the bell of the stethoscope. S_3 usually has a dull, thudlike quality. Its timing is closely related to S_2, which is heard just after the T wave; S_3 follows S_2 by less than 0.2 seconds.

4. Because S_3 is associated with blood volume and velocity, it can be intensified by maneuvers that increase stroke volume,

such as elevating the patient's legs from a recumbent position or having the patient exercise briefly or cough several times. Placing the patient in the partial left lateral recumbent position may enhance your ability to auscultate and palpate an S_3.

5. An S_3 sometimes originates in the right ventricle instead of the left; when it does, it's always considered abnormal. A right-sided S_3 is heard best over the third, fourth, and fifth intercostal spaces along the left sternal border or over the epigastric area. It's more prominent during inspiration because of increased blood flow into the right ventricle.

6. By the end of diastole, the ventricles are nearly full; atrial contraction further stretches and fills the ventricles. The vibrations caused by this filling and stretching in late diastole generate an additional heart sound, S_4, sometimes called an atrial diastolic gallop.

7. S_4 is usually heard best near the heart's apex over the mitral area; occasionally, it's also palpable over this area. In some patients, it's faint in intensity and difficult to hear, but in others it's loud and easily heard. S_4 is relatively short in duration and may occur only intermittently, during every third or fourth heartbeat. It has a low pitch that's heard best using the bell of the stethoscope, and it has a thudlike quality. Its timing is presystolic: S_4 precedes S_1 and occurs during the P-R interval.

8. To enhance S_4, place the patient in the partial left lateral recumbent position, which brings the heart closer to the chest wall.

9. An abnormal S_4 is almost always associated with increased mean left atrial pressure caused by a noncompliant left ventricle. This auscultatory finding is heard in patients with hypertension, hypertrophic cardiomyopathy, cardiomyopathies, or ischemic heart disease and during or after an acute myocardial infarction. When an S_4 is heard in a patient with hypertension, the systolic blood pressure usually exceeds 160 mm Hg or the

diastolic pressure exceeds 100 mm Hg. An abnormal S_4 can also accompany volume overload conditions, such as hyperthyroidism, severe anemia, and sudden severe mitral regurgitation.

10. Normally, S_4 precedes S_1 by an appreciable interval that correlates with the P-R interval on the ECG. However, in patients with first-degree AV block, the P wave occurs early in diastole, and S_4 may occur during the early rapid diastolic filling period. Likewise, in tachycardia, S_4 may be superimposed on S_3 during early rapid filling. Should either condition exist, the S_4 fuses with S_3 to become a single diastolic filling sound called a summation gallop, which may be louder than S_4, S_3, or S_1.

6 Other diastolic and systolic sounds

1. An OS is usually heard best near the heart's apex over the mitral area or just medial to it. Its intensity varies among patients, and it's usually easy to hear during auscultation. An OS has a short duration. It has a high pitch that's heard best using the diaphragm of the stethoscope, and it has a sharp, snaplike quality. Its timing is closely related to S_2: an OS occurs early in ventricular diastole, just after the stenotic mitral valve opens.

2. One characteristic of an OS that helps distinguish it from P_2 is its timing: the A_2-P_2 interval is normally shorter than the A_2-OS interval. Also, when the patient stands, the A_2-P_2 interval narrows, whereas the A_2-OS interval widens. Another characteristic is that the A_2-OS interval remains constant throughout respiration, whereas the A_2-P_2 interval normally widens during inspiration and narrows during expiration. During inspiration, three distinct sounds can usually be heard over the pulmonic area; therefore, the sequence must be A_2, P_2, OS. In contrast, during expiration, the A_2-P_2 interval narrows or fuses, forming one sound. This creates an S_2-OS interval. Finally, P_2 usually isn't heard over the

mitral area, so if you hear a split S_2 over this area, it is likely to be an S_2 and an OS.

3. One characteristic of an OS that helps distinguish it from an S_3 is its timing: the A_2-S_3 interval is usually longer than the A_2-OS interval. Also, S_3 is a low-frequency sound that's heard best over the mitral area using the bell of the stethoscope. In contrast, an OS produces a high-frequency sound that's more widely transmitted across the precordium and is heard best using the diaphragm of the stethoscope.

   Another characteristic of an OS is that its intensity usually isn't affected by having the patient stand, whereas S_3 intensity can be decreased by standing. If the OS is affected, it's intensified. Another way to differentiate S_3 from an OS is by listening for respiratory changes. An S_3 is usually louder during expiration than during inspiration and, in many patients, is palpable; an OS doesn't vary in intensity with respiration. Finally, if the murmur typically heard in patients with mitral stenosis is present, you can confirm that the sound is an OS.

4. A systolic ejection sound (ES) is usually a brief, high-frequency sound that's heard best using the diaphragm of the stethoscope. It may be heard near the heart's base over the aortic or pulmonic area, over Erb point, or near the apex over the mitral area. A systolic ES occurs just after the QRS complex on the ECG waveform.

5. A PES is usually heard best near the heart's base over the pulmonic area. Its intensity is soft but may be equal to or greater than that of S_1. A PES has a short duration. It has a high pitch that's heard best using the diaphragm of the stethoscope, and it has a sharp, or clicklike, quality. Its timing is closely related to S_1: it occurs early in ventricular systole, just after the opening of a stenotic pulmonic valve, and is heard just after the QRS complex.

6. An AES is heard best near the heart's apex over the mitral area, near the heart's base over the aortic area, or over Erb point. To enhance the sound, have the patient sit up and lean forward. The intensity of an AES is soft but may be equal to or greater than that of S_1. To distinguish it from a split S_2, ask the patient to take a deep breath and hold it.

   An AES has a short duration. It has a high pitch that's heard best using the diaphragm of the stethoscope, and it has a sharp, or clicklike, quality. Its timing is closely related to S_1. An AES occurs early in ventricular systole, just after the opening of a stenotic aortic valve, and is heard just after the QRS complex on the ECG waveform.

7. Certain characteristics help to distinguish an AES from other heart sounds. One characteristic is that an AES radiates more than a PES. Another characteristic is that a split S_1 heard over the mitral area is likely to be an M_1 and an AES.

   You can differentiate an AES from an S_4 by remembering that S_4 is heard best over the mitral area using the bell of the stethoscope and is commonly accompanied by a palpable, presystolic apical bulge. Also, an S_4 is intensified by maneuvers that increase left atrial pressures, such as brief exercise, squatting, or coughing. An AES is unaffected by these maneuvers.

8. A midsystolic click (MSC) occurs when the prolapsed mitral valve's leaflets and chordae tendineae tense. The anterior leaflet, the posterior leaflet, or both can prolapse, causing a balloon backup into the left atrium.

9. An MSC is usually heard best over the tricuspid area and near the heart's apex over the mitral area. Its intensity is equal to or greater than that of S_1. An MSC has a short duration. It has a high pitch that's heard best using the diaphragm of the stethoscope, and it has a clicklike quality. The click's timing varies: it can occur in early systole, midsystole, or late systole.

An MSC can be heard during the Q-T interval on the ECG waveform.

10. The timing of an MSC is affected by various maneuvers, such as having the patient stand or perform Valsalva maneuver. Such maneuvers result in reduced left ventricular filling and cause the MSC to be heard closer to S_1. The MSC may even merge with S_1 and disappear completely. Increasing the left ventricular volume by raising the legs from a recumbent position or squatting delays the click. This maneuver may also cause the prolapse not to occur and the MSC to be diminished or inaudible. Sometimes an MSC is accompanied by a late systolic crescendo murmur or the characteristic holosystolic murmur of mitral regurgitation. An MSC may also be caused by some extracardiac conditions, such as pleuropericardial adhesions.

7 Murmur fundamentals

1. The terms used to describe a specific characteristic are determined primarily by the volume and speed of the jet of blood as it moves through the heart.

2. A murmur's location is the anatomic area on the chest wall where the murmur is heard best and is usually also the murmur's point of maximum intensity. This area usually correlates with the underlying location of the valve that's responsible for producing the murmur.

3. A murmur's sound may be transmitted to the chamber or vessel where the turbulent blood flow occurs. This phenomenon, known as radiation, occurs because the direction of blood flow determines sound transmission. Murmurs radiate in either forward or backward direction.

4. Intensity refers to the murmur's loudness.

5. To document a murmur's intensity, most health care professionals use a six-point graded scale, with 1 being the faintest intensity and 6 being the loudest. A grade 1 murmur is faint and is barely heard through the stethoscope. A grade 2 murmur is also faint but is usually heard as soon as the stethoscope is placed on the chest wall. A grade 3 murmur is easily heard and is described as moderately loud. A grade 4 murmur is loud and is usually associated with a palpable vibration known as a thrill. It may also radiate in the direction of blood flow. A grade 5 murmur is loud enough to be heard with only an edge of the stethoscope touching the chest wall; it's almost always accompanied by a thrill and radiation. A grade 6 murmur is so loud that it can be heard with the stethoscope close to, but not touching, the chest wall; it's always accompanied by a thrill and it radiates to distant structures.

6. A murmur's duration is the length of time the murmur is heard during systole or diastole; it may be described as long or short.

7. A murmur's pitch, or frequency, varies from high-pitched to low-pitched.

8. A murmur's quality is determined by the combination of frequencies that produces the sound. It's typically described as harsh, rough, musical, scratchy, squeaky, rumbling, or blowing.

9. A murmur's timing refers to when the murmur occurs in the cardiac cycle. This means that the onset, duration, and end of the murmur are described in relation to systole and diastole. Murmurs are further classified according to their timing within the phases of the cardiac cycle. For example, a murmur can be described as holosystolic (present throughout systole); early systolic, midsystolic, or late systolic; or early diastolic, middiastolic, or late diastolic.

10. A murmur's configuration refers to the shape of a murmur's sound as recorded on a phonocardiogram. The configuration is usually defined by changes in the murmur's intensity during systole or diastole and is determined by blood flow pressure gradients.

8 Systolic murmurs

1. An SEM is usually heard best along the left sternal border and sometimes over the aortic and mitral areas. Its intensity is

usually soft (less than a grade 3/6), and its duration is short. It has a medium pitch that's heard best using the diaphragm of the stethoscope. The quality of an SEM varies. Its timing is early systolic; it ends well before a normal S_2 split. It's heard after the QRS complex on the ECG waveform. An SEM has a crescendo–decrescendo configuration.

2. A supravalvular pulmonic stenosis murmur is usually heard over much of the thorax. Its intensity and duration are variable. It has a medium pitch that's heard best using the diaphragm of the stethoscope, and it has a harsh quality. Its timing is systolic: it begins after S_1 and ends before a normal S_2 split. On the ECG waveform, the murmur begins just after the QRS complex begins and ends just before the T wave ends. It has a crescendo–decrescendo configuration that's occasionally continuous.

3. A pulmonic valvular stenosis murmur is heard best near the heart's base over the pulmonic area. It commonly radiates toward the left neck or the left shoulder. The murmur's intensity is usually soft, but it will become louder as the stenosis becomes more severe. Its duration is short, but this too will increase as the stenosis worsens. It has a medium pitch that's heard best using the diaphragm of the stethoscope, and it has a harsh quality. The murmur's timing is midsystolic: it ends before a normal S_2 split. In the ECG waveform, it begins after the QRS complex and ends before the T wave ends. It has a crescendo–decrescendo configuration. A mild pulmonic valvular stenosis murmur is shaped like a diamond; a severe pulmonic valvular stenosis murmur is shaped like a kite.

4. A subvalvular pulmonic stenosis murmur is usually heard best over the pulmonic area and over Erb point; it commonly radiates toward the left side of the neck, the left shoulder, or both. Its intensity is usually soft but becomes louder as the stenosis worsens. Its duration, which is

short, also increases as the stenosis worsens. The murmur has a medium pitch that's heard best using the diaphragm of the stethoscope, and it has a harsh quality. Its timing is midsystolic: it starts after S_1 and ends before a normal S_2 split. In the ECG waveform, the murmur begins after the QRS complex and ends before the end of the T wave. This murmur isn't initiated by a pulmonic ejection sound. It has a crescendo–decrescendo configuration.

5. A supravalvular aortic stenosis murmur is usually heard best near the heart's base over the right first intercostal space, over the aortic area, and over the suprasternal notch. It may radiate toward the right side of the neck, the right shoulder, or both. Its intensity, typically a 3/6 to 4/6, decreases in patients with left-sided heart failure. Its duration increases as the stenosis worsens. It has a medium pitch that can be heard equally well using the diaphragm or bell of the stethoscope. The murmur has a rough quality. Its timing is midsystolic: it ends before a normal S_2 split. It isn't associated with an aortic ejection sound. On the ECG waveform, it begins after the QRS complex and ends before the end of the T wave. The murmur has a crescendo–decrescendo configuration.

6. An aortic valvular stenosis murmur is usually heard best near the heart's base over the aortic area, over Erb point, near the heart's apex over the mitral area, or over the suprasternal notch. The murmur may radiate toward the right side of the neck, the right shoulder, or both. A thrill may be palpable over the aortic area and neck. The intensity, typically a grade 3/6 to 4/6, decreases in patients with left-sided heart failure. The murmur's duration increases as stenosis worsens.

An aortic valvular stenosis murmur has a medium pitch that's heard equally well using the diaphragm or bell of the stethoscope. The murmur's quality is rough and may become harsher and louder as stenosis worsens. Its timing is midsystolic. An aortic ejection sound (AES), when present, is heard shortly after S_1; the AES is followed by the murmur, which ends before a normal S_2 split. In the ECG waveform, the murmur begins after the QRS complex and ends before the end of the T wave. It has a crescendo–decrescendo configuration. As the stenosis worsens, valve motion is reduced and the aortic component of the S_2 disappears.

7. A subvalvular aortic stenosis murmur is usually heard best near the heart's apex over the mitral and tricuspid areas. It doesn't usually radiate toward the base, right side of the neck, or the right shoulder. Its intensity, typically a grade 3/6 to 4/6, will increase as stenosis worsens; its duration varies. The murmur has a medium pitch that's heard equally well with the bell or diaphragm of the stethoscope. Its quality can be harsh or rough. This murmur's timing is midsystolic: it peaks in midsystole and ends before a normal S_2 split, a delayed A_2, or a paradoxical S_2 split. On the ECG waveform, it begins after the QRS complex and ends before the end of the T wave. The murmur has a crescendo–decrescendo configuration.

8. A tricuspid regurgitation murmur is usually heard best over the tricuspid area; in some patients, it's heard only during inspiration. The murmur may radiate to the right of the sternum. Its usually soft intensity may increase during deep inspiration. The murmur's duration is long. It has a medium pitch that's heard best using the diaphragm of the stethoscope, and it has a scratchy or blowing quality. The murmur's timing is systolic: it lasts from S_1 to P_2. On the ECG waveform, the murmur begins just after the QRS complex and ends after the T wave. It's holosystolic and plateau-shaped.

9. A holosystolic mitral regurgitation murmur is usually heard best near the heart's apex over the mitral area. The sound may radiate to the axillae or posteriorly over the lung bases. Its intensity varies and usually is unaffected by respiration; however, it may be somewhat diminished during inspiration. The murmur has a long duration. It has a medium to high pitch that's heard best using the diaphragm of the stethoscope. The murmur may be accompanied by a systolic apical thrill. Its quality is blowing, and its timing is systolic—from S_1 to S_2. On the ECG waveform, it's heard from just after the QRS complex to the end of the T wave. The murmur is holosystolic and plateau-shaped.

10. An acute mitral regurgitation murmur is usually heard best near the heart's apex over the mitral area. Its intensity is usually loud (a grade 4/6 to 6/6 if the murmur results from rupture of the chordae tendineae). It's accompanied by a systolic thrill. The murmur's duration is medium long. It has a high pitch that's heard best using the diaphragm of the stethoscope, and it has a musical quality. Its timing is systolic: it begins with M_1 and ends with or before A_2. On the ECG waveform, the murmur begins just after the QRS complex and ends just after the T wave. It's commonly holosystolic and wedge-shaped (the wedge shape has a steeper decrescendo configuration).

11. A mitral valve prolapse murmur is usually heard best near the heart's apex over the mitral area. Its intensity is usually soft (a grade 2/6 to 3/6), and its duration is short. It has a high pitch that's heard best with the diaphragm of the stethoscope. The murmur has a musical quality; when loud, it's sometimes described as a whoop or honk. Its timing is usually late systolic but can sometimes be holosystolic. In the ECG waveform, the murmur coincides with the T wave and ends just after the T wave. It has a crescendo or crescendo–decrescendo configuration.

9 Diastolic murmurs

1. An early diastolic aortic regurgitation murmur is usually heard best near the heart's base over the aortic and pulmonic

areas, over Erb point, and near the heart's apex over the mitral area. Because of its usually soft intensity, it's heard best in a quiet environment. The murmur can last throughout most of diastole. It has a high pitch that's heard best using the diaphragm of the stethoscope, and it has a blowing or musical quality. Its timing is diastolic, beginning with A_2. On the ECG waveform, the murmur begins after the T wave ends and ends just before the QRS complex. It has a decrescendo configuration.

2. This murmur can be enhanced by having the patient sit down, lean forward, and hold his breath after expiration or perform maneuvers that increase aortic diastolic pressure, such as squatting or performing handgrip exercises.

3. An Austin Flint murmur is usually heard best near the heart's apex over the mitral area. Its intensity is usually soft. It has a low pitch that's heard best using the bell of the stethoscope. The murmur has a rumbling quality. Its timing is confined to middiastole and presystole. It's heard just before the QRS complex on the ECG waveform. The murmur has a presystolic crescendo configuration; its middiastolic component has a crescendo–decrescendo configuration.

4. A Graham Steell murmur secondary to pulmonary hypertension is usually heard best along the left sternal border over the third and fourth intercostal spaces. It isn't transmitted to the right sternum. Its intensity is usually loud, and its duration varies. The murmur has a high pitch that's heard best using the diaphragm of the stethoscope, and it has a blowing quality. Its timing is early diastolic, beginning with a loud P_2. Sometimes an ejection sound can be heard. The murmur is heard after the end of the T wave in the ECG waveform and usually doesn't extend to S_1. It has a decrescendo configuration.

5. The normal pressure pulmonic valve murmur is usually heard best along the left sternal border over the third and fourth

intercostal spaces. It isn't transmitted to the right sternum. Its intensity is soft and its duration brief. The murmur has a low pitch that's heard best using the bell of the stethoscope. It has a rumbling quality and its timing is early diastolic to middiastolic. It begins shortly after P_2 is heard. On the ECG waveform, it begins after the T wave and ends before the P wave. The murmur has a crescendo–decrescendo configuration.

6. A normal pressure pulmonic valve murmur is intensified during inspiration.

7. Scarring and calcification of the valve create a funnel-shaped opening between the left atrium and left ventricle. A mitral stenosis murmur starts with an opening snap (OS) after A_2 and isovolumetric relaxation; this OS is an important diagnostic feature of mitral stenosis. The murmur is produced by rapid, turbulent blood flow through a rigid, narrowed mitral valve opening. Turbulence increases just before systole; this gives the murmur its characteristic presystolic crescendo.

8. A mitral stenosis murmur is usually heard best near the heart's apex over the mitral area. Its intensity and duration vary. It has a low pitch that's heard best using the bell of the stethoscope and a rumbling quality that has been compared to thunder. The timing of a mitral stenosis murmur is diastolic: it begins after A_2 with an OS and ends with a loud M_1. However, stenosis severity affects the murmur's duration. On the ECG waveform, the murmur begins just after the T wave and ends during the QRS complex. It has a crescendo–decrescendo configuration. In patients with normal sinus rhythm, the presystolic component has a crescendo configuration.

9. A mitral stenosis murmur is heard best with the patient in a partial left lateral recumbent position. It can be intensified by maneuvers that increase cardiac output, such as having the patient exercise for a few minutes, raise his legs from a recumbent position, or cough several times.

10. A tricuspid stenosis murmur is usually heard best over the tricuspid area. Its usually soft intensity increases during inspiration and fades or disappears during expiration. The murmur's duration varies. It has a low pitch that's heard best using the bell of the stethoscope while the patient is in the partial left lateral recumbent position. The murmur has a rumbling quality. Its timing is middiastolic to late diastolic: it ends just before S_1. An opening snap may be heard. In the ECG waveform, the murmur begins just after the T wave and ends just before the QRS complex. In patients with normal sinus rhythm, it has a late diastolic crescendo or crescendo–decrescendo configuration.

10 Continuous murmurs

1. Continuous murmurs are generated by rapid blood flow through arteries or veins or by shunting. Shunting occurs when an abnormal communication is created between the high-pressure arterial system and the low-pressure venous system. The murmurs begin in systole and persist, without interruption, through S_2 into diastole.

2. A normal cervical venous hum is caused by rapid downward blood flow through the jugular veins in the lower part of the neck.

3. A cervical venous hum murmur is heard best over the right supraclavicular fossa when the patient is sitting and his head is turned to the left. It has a faint intensity that increases during diastole. The murmur has a long duration: it lasts throughout the cardiac cycle. Its high pitch is heard best using the diaphragm of the stethoscope. Its quality is soft and its timing continuous. The hum is louder between S_2 and S_1. The murmur has a plateau shape in systole and a crescendo–decrescendo configuration in diastole.

4. A patent ductus arteriosus (PDA) murmur is heard best over the left first intercostal space, over the pulmonic area, and below the left clavicle. Its intensity is faint when the murmur is limited to this area. If the murmur is loud, the systolic component may be heard along the left sternal border and sometimes over the mitral area. A loud PDA murmur may radiate to the back between the scapulae. A PDA murmur has a long duration. Its intensity varies, roughly correlating with the ductus size; typically, the murmur reaches maximum intensity late in systole and then fades during diastole. A PDA murmur has a high pitch that's heard equally well using the bell or diaphragm of the stethoscope. It has a rough, machinery-like quality, and its timing is continuous. It begins with—or shortly after—a normal S_1 and disappears just before the next S_1. Because the murmur peaks in late systole, S_2 may be difficult to hear. S_2 may be paradoxically split if the left ventricular ejection time is prolonged. An S_3 may be heard over the mitral area. The murmur has a crescendo–decrescendo configuration.

5. Exercise can increase the intensity and duration of a PDA murmur.

6. To differentiate between a PDA murmur and a cervical venous hum murmur, remember that the hum is loudest above the clavicle, is usually heard better on the right, and can be obliterated by pressing on the jugular vein or placing the patient in a supine position. The venous hum is truly continuous and is usually louder during diastole.

11 Other auscultatory sounds

1. The murmur generated by an aortic ball-in-cage valve prosthesis is usually heard best near the apex over the mitral and aortic areas and along the left sternal border. Its intensity is usually loud and easy to hear, and its duration varies. It has a medium pitch that's heard best using the diaphragm of the stethoscope. The murmur has a crunchy, harsh quality. Its timing is midsystolic. The interval between the aortic closing click and P_2 is similar to the normal A_2-P_2 interval, and it normally widens during inspiration. The murmur has a crescendo–decrescendo configuration.

2. The murmur generated by an aortic tilting-disk valve prosthesis is usually heard best near the apex over the mitral and aortic areas and along the left sternal border. Its intensity is usually soft (grade 2/6) and its duration short. It has a medium pitch that's heard best using the diaphragm of the stethoscope. The murmur has a rough or harsh quality. Its timing is systolic. The interval between the aortic closing click and P_2 is similar to the normal A_2-P_2 interval, and it widens during inspiration. The murmur has a crescendo–decrescendo configuration.

3. The murmur generated by an aortic bileaflet valve prosthesis is usually heard best near the apex over the mitral and aortic areas and along the left sternal border with the patient in the left lateral decubitus position. Its intensity is usually soft (grade 2/6) and its duration short. It has a medium pitch that's heard best using the diaphragm of the stethoscope. The murmur has a rough or harsh quality, and its timing is systolic. The interval between the aortic closing click and P_2 is similar to the normal A_2-P_2 interval, and it widens during inspiration. The murmur has a crescendo–decrescendo configuration.

4. The murmur generated by an aortic porcine valve prosthesis is usually heard best near the apex over the mitral and aortic areas and along the left sternal border. Its intensity is usually soft (grade 2/6) and its duration short. It has a medium pitch that's heard best using the diaphragm of the stethoscope. The murmur has a rough or harsh quality, and its timing is systolic. The interval between the aortic closing sound and P_2 is similar to the normal A_2-P_2 interval, and it widens during inspiration. The murmur has a crescendo–decrescendo configuration.

5. With a mitral ball-in-cage valve, M_1 is loud and higher in frequency. A mitral opening click follows a normal S_2.

6. A normally functioning mitral tilting-disk valve prosthesis replaces M_1 with a mitral closing click. This closing click is always distinctly audible and high-pitched; its maximum intensity is located near the apex over the mitral area.

7. In a systolic murmur generated by the mitral bileaflet valve, the first sound is replaced by a higher-pitched sound. The mitral opening click, though rarely heard, follows a normal S_2.

8. The systolic murmur generated by a mitral porcine valve prosthesis is usually heard best near the apex over the mitral area and sounds like a normal M_1.

9. A pericardial friction rub is usually heard best—and is sometimes palpable—over the tricuspid and xyphoid areas. It's usually loud and may get louder during inspiration. The rub has a high pitch that's heard best using the diaphragm of the stethoscope, and it has a grating or scratchy quality. It's usually heard during each cardiac cycle. It has a systolic component and an early and late diastolic component. The diastolic component may last for only a few hours.

10. The noises produced by mediastinal crunch are usually heard best along the left sternal border with the patient in the sitting position. The noises have a crunching quality, which may become louder during inspiration.

BREATH SOUNDS

12 The respiratory system and auscultation

1. The respiratory system's primary function is the exchange of oxygen (O_2) and carbon dioxide (CO_2) between the alveoli and the pulmonary circulation.

2. The mainstem bronchi enter the lungs at the hila, where the lung tissue attaches to the mediastinum. The bronchi course downward and immediately divide into lobar bronchi, which subdivide into segmental bronchi. The airways continue to systematically branch, narrow, shorten, and increase in number toward the lung

periphery. They divide about 25 times before ultimately opening into the terminal, or respiratory, bronchioles. The terminal bronchioles, which have a few alveoli budding from their walls, branch into the alveolar ducts, which are completely lined with alveoli.

3. The lung's apex (superior aspect) is located near the clavicle, and its base (inferior aspect) is located near the diaphragm.

4. During inspiration, the diaphragm and intercostal muscles are activated. Diaphragmatic contraction flattens the domed diaphragm and expands the lower rib cage, forcing the abdominal contents downward and out, thus increasing the longitudinal lung size. Intercostal muscle contraction stabilizes the rib cage and moves it outward and upward. The posterior cricoarytenoid muscle contracts to open the glottis. As the thorax expands, intrapleural pressures become subatmospheric, resulting in lung expansion and decreased intrapulmonary pressures. Inspired air flows from higher atmospheric pressure into the airways. At the end of inspiration, diaphragmatic movement declines and the air inflow gradually slows.

During expiration, the thorax and the elastic recoil force of the lungs return to their resting positions, increasing intrapleural pressures. This increased pressure forces air to flow out of the lower and upper airways. At the end of expiration, during quiet breathing, all muscles are relaxed and the diaphragm has returned to its resting position.

5. During normal breathing in the upright position, air movement (ventilation) is greatest in the lung bases or dependent lung regions. Because of the pull of gravity, the alveoli in the lung bases collapse to a smaller size during expiration than do the alveoli in the lung apices. During inspiration, the alveoli in the lung bases open more easily, causing ventilation in the bases to be greater than in the apices.

Blood perfusion in the lungs is also gravity-dependent; the dependent lung regions receive a larger proportion of the cardiac output than the nondependent regions.

6. The lung apices extend 1¼" to 1½" (2 to 4 cm) above the clavicles. The trachea bifurcates at the level of the sternal angle, the junction between the manubrium and the body of the sternum. The ribs and intercostal spaces provide precise horizontal landmarks to describe the location of breath sounds; the second rib and second intercostal space serve as reference points.

Vertical landmark lines on the anterior chest wall surface include the midclavicular lines and the midsternal line. The right and left midclavicular lines extend downward from the center of each clavicle. The midsternal line bisects the sternum. The right lung base crosses the sixth rib at the right midclavicular line, and the left lung base crosses the seventh rib at the left midclavicular line.

7. The anterior axillary line extends downward from the anterior axillary fold, the midaxillary line extends downward from the apex of the axilla, and the posterior axillary line extends downward from the posterior axillary fold.

8. Bony structures underlying the posterior chest wall surface also provide landmarks to locate breath sounds. The scapulae's inferior borders, located at about the same level as the seventh rib, serve as reference points. The numbered thoracic vertebrae provide horizontal landmarks. Landmark lines on the posterior chest wall surface provide vertical reference points. The midscapular lines extend downward from the inferior angle of each scapula, and the vertebral line extends downward over the vertebrae.

9. During auscultation, press the diaphragm of the stethoscope firmly against the patient's chest wall over the intercostal spaces. Try not to listen directly over bone; never listen through

clothing, which impedes or alters sound transmission.

10. If the patient is alert and healthy, begin auscultation with the patient sitting upright and leaning slightly forward with his hands grasping his elbows to separate the scapulae. Position yourself behind the patient. Ask the patient to breathe through an open mouth, slightly deeper and faster than usual, through several respiratory cycles. Place the diaphragm of the stethoscope over the left lung apex, and listen for at least one complete respiratory cycle. Then move the diaphragm to the same site over the right lung. Compare the breath sounds heard over these same locations. Continue in this manner, making contralateral comparisons at each auscultatory site.

13 Introduction to breath sounds

1. Breath sounds are produced by airflow patterns, by associated pressure changes within the airways, and by solid tissue vibrations within the lungs.

2. Sounds heard over the trachea and large airways are characterized as high-pitched, harsh, loud, and tubular (hollow) with a long expiratory phase. These sounds are thought to reflect the turbulent airflow patterns in the first divisions of the large airways. Sounds heard over other chest wall areas are softer and have a shorter expiratory phase.

3. During rapid or turbulent airflow, air molecules move randomly, colliding against airway walls and each other. They may move across or against the general direction of airflow. The colliding air molecules produce rapid pressure changes within the airway, and these rapid pressure changes produce sounds. Turbulent airflow occurs in the trachea, mainstem bronchi, and other larger airways.

4. As airflow is forced to change directions abruptly in the branching airways, the airstream separates into layers and moves at different velocities. The shearing force of high-velocity airstreams, along with slower airstreams, precipitates opposing circular airflows, or vortices. This airflow pattern generates sounds as the flow of air carries the vortices downstream.

5. In the terminal or small airways and respiratory bronchioles, airflow is slow and laminar. No abrupt changes in pressure or airway wall movements occur to generate sound. Consequently, air movement in these areas produces no sound.

6. Frequency, measured in hertz, refers to the number of vibrations occurring per unit of time. The term *pitch* is used to describe sound frequency. High-pitched sounds have higher frequencies; low-pitched sounds, lower frequencies. Intensity is the loudness or softness of the vibrations producing breath sounds. It can be measured electronically by recording amplitude. Intensity is affected by the type of vibrating structure producing the sound, the distance the sound travels, and the transmission pathway. The duration of the vibrations that produce breath sounds can be measured in milliseconds. However, the human ear perceives sounds during auscultation as long or short and as continuous or discontinuous.

7. The tracheal and bronchial sounds, produced by turbulent airflow, are loud and can be heard throughout inspiration and expiration over the trachea and mainstem bronchi. Normal breath sounds heard over other chest wall areas are faint and can be heard throughout inspiration and at the beginning of expiration.

8. Voice sounds auscultated over the chest wall are called bronchophony. In a healthy individual, bronchophony is similar to voice sounds heard through the neck. Voice sounds transmitted through the chest wall that have selectively amplified higher-pitched frequencies are called egophony. High-pitched, distinct, whispered sounds transmitted through airless, consolidated lung tissue are called whispered pectoriloquy.

9. Adventitious sounds are added sounds that are heard with abnormal breath sounds. They're classified into two categories: crackles and wheezes.

10. Location, intensity, duration, and pitch are the four characteristics used to describe breath sounds.

14 Breath sounds heard in healthy individuals

1. Normal breath sounds are broadly defined as breathing heard through the chest wall of a healthy individual.

2. Three variables affect the normal sounds heard during auscultation: the distance between the source of the sound and the chest wall, the path of sound transmission, and the sound's location.

3. Normal breath sounds are produced by airflow patterns, by associated pressure changes within the airways, and by solid tissue vibrations.

4. Tracheal and mainstem bronchi breath sounds are heard over the chest wall on either side of the sternum from the second intercostal space to the fourth intercostal space anteriorly and along the vertebral column from the third intercostal space to the sixth intercostal space posteriorly. These sounds have a variable pitch and a loud intensity that's heard best using the diaphragm of the stethoscope. They're heard throughout inspiration and expiration.

5. These normal breath sounds are heard throughout the chest anteriorly, posteriorly, and laterally. Their duration varies, depending on their location, but inspiration is usually followed immediately by a shorter expiration. The sounds have a low pitch that can be heard using either the diaphragm or bell of the stethoscope.

6. Variations in intensity are usually related to airflow patterns and to the distribution of ventilation throughout the lungs. During inspiration, with the patient in the upright position, air flows initially into the lung apices, then into the lung bases (the dependent areas) after the small airways

reopen; therefore, the intensity will probably be greater in the apices than in the bases. During normal breathing, this change in intensity may not always be audible.

7. The intensity may increase during systole because ventricular contraction allows the surrounding lung tissue to expand more fully, increasing turbulent airflow to that region and intensifying the inspiratory sounds. Conversely, the intensity may decrease during diastole because ventricular expansion of the heart compresses adjacent lung tissue, reducing airflow to that region.

8. Normal breath sounds heard at the mouth are thought to be produced by turbulent airflow occurring below the glottis and before the terminal airways. In healthy individuals, breath sounds at the mouth provide baseline data that can be useful later when evaluating noisy or paradoxically quiet breath sounds.

15 Bronchial breath sounds

1. When lung tissue between the central airways and the chest wall becomes airless because of conditions that increase lung density, transmission of breath sounds from large airways is enhanced.

2. Breath sounds are enhanced over an area of increased lung density because little high-frequency sound is lost through attenuation or filtration. As lung tissue density increases the impedance between the fluid-filled lung tissue and the pleurae and chest wall, these three media become well-matched. This match decreases the normal filtering of high-frequency sounds. Consequently, the breath sounds are transmitted more readily to the chest wall surface and are louder and more tubular than normal breath sounds heard over the same chest wall area.

3. The conditions associated with bronchial breath sounds include consolidation, atelectasis, and fibrosis.

4. Clinical findings vary, depending on the location of the consolidated area and the

causative agent. However, when classic consolidation is present, decreased chest wall movement and a dull percussion note are apparent over the affected area.

5. Bronchial breathing is heard over a dense, airless upper lobe, even without a patent bronchus, because the upper lobe surfaces are in direct contact with the trachea and loud tracheal breath sounds are transmitted directly to the dense, airless upper lobe tissues. In contrast, bronchial breath sounds are heard over a dense, airless lower lobe only when the bronchi are patent because sound isn't transmitted directly to the airless lower lobe tissues.

6. Bronchial breath sounds heard over a consolidated area are high-pitched and have the typical hollow, or tubular, quality of normal central airway breath sounds. They remain audible during both expiration and inspiration, but the expiratory sounds are longer and louder when the patient is sitting up. The I:E ratio is 1:2. These sounds may be auscultated using either the bell or diaphragm of the stethoscope.

7. Atelectasis, the incomplete expansion of a lung area, is thought to result from uncleared secretions that become thick, occluding the airway, or from hypoventilation.

8. Bronchial breath sounds heard over an atelectatic area are high-pitched and have the typical hollow, or tubular, quality of normal central airway breath sounds. They're audible throughout inspiration and expiration. When the patient is in the supine position, the inspiratory and expiratory sounds are equal in duration and intensity. The I:E ratio is 1:1. These sounds can be heard equally well using either the bell or diaphragm of the stethoscope.

9. Bronchial breath sounds heard over a fibrotic area have the typical hollow, or tubular, quality of normal central airway breath sounds. They're audible throughout inspiration and expiration. When the patient is in the upright position, the breath sounds become progressively louder during inspiration and become both louder and longer during expiration. The I:E ratio is 1:1 to 1:2. These bronchial breath sounds are high-pitched and are heard equally well using either the diaphragm or bell of the stethoscope.

16 Abnormal voice sounds

1. Voice sounds are produced by vibrations of the vocal cords as air from the lungs passes over them. The resonance of the mouth, nasopharynx, and paranasal sinuses helps to amplify these sounds.

2. Transmitted voice sounds are normally heard as a low-pitched, unintelligible mumble over healthy lung and pleural surfaces because most of the vowels are filtered out.

3. Voice sounds are heard distinctly over consolidated or atelectatic lung tissue areas because less filtering takes place, enhancing transmission.

4. Bronchophony can be heard anywhere over the anterior, lateral, and posterior chest wall surfaces. It's commonly heard over dense, airless lung tissue in the upper lobes, such as a consolidated area.

5. The patient is asked to repeat the words "ninety-nine" several times. Over healthy lung tissue, the words are unintelligible; however, over a consolidated area, the high-frequency sounds are easily understood as words.

6. Whispered pectoriloquy can be heard anywhere over the anterior or posterior chest wall surfaces over dense, airless lung tissue, typically over an area of consolidation or atelectasis.

7. Egophony, a voice sound that has a nasal or bleating quality when heard over the chest wall, is produced over consolidated and atelectatic areas because impedance matching enhances breath sound transmission in such areas. It's also detectable over the upper border of large pleural effusions.

8. Egophony can be heard anywhere over the anterior, posterior, or lateral chest wall surfaces over a consolidated or atelectatic area.

9. The patient is asked to repeat the letter "E" several times. Over healthy lung tissue, the letter sounds as it normally does; over the consolidated area, it sounds like "A-aay" and has a high-pitched, nasal quality.

10. Bronchial breath sounds, bronchophony, whispered pectoriloquy, and egophony are typical in patients with consolidation.

17 Absent and diminished breath sounds

1. Breath sounds are diminished or eliminated by conditions that limit airflow into lung segments. Slow inspiratory airflow rates decrease breath sound amplitude because less air movement occurs, resulting in less turbulent airflow. Diminished or absent breath sounds can also occur when breath sounds are reflected at the visceral and parietal pleurae because of an impedance mismatch.

2. During normal breathing in the upright position, a certain amount of air flows through the airways during inspiration and expiration; the distribution of ventilation is greater in dependent lung regions because more respiratory movement occurs. During shallow breathing, less respiratory movement occurs; consequently, less air flows through the airways during inspiration and expiration. Because of this reduced airflow, turbulence is decreased and breath sounds are diminished.

3. If a lobar or segmental bronchus becomes obstructed, as in a patient who has aspirated a foreign object, airflow ceases distal to the obstruction; therefore, breath sounds will be absent over the area distal to the obstruction. If a mainstem bronchus is obstructed, breath sounds will be absent throughout the affected lung.

4. Breath sounds heard over a pneumothorax are significantly diminished or absent because of acoustical mismatching of the air-filled lung and the collection of air in the pleural space.

5. Diminished or absent breath sounds resulting from a pneumothorax can occur anywhere over the anterior, posterior, and lateral chest wall surfaces, depending on the location and size of the pneumothorax. Normal breath sounds are heard on the contralateral side over healthy lung tissue, and breath sounds are absent over the pneumothorax. If diminished breath sounds are heard, they have a low pitch that's heard using either the bell or diaphragm of the stethoscope.

6. Diminished or absent breath sounds resulting from a pleural effusion may be heard anywhere over the anterior, posterior, or lateral chest wall surfaces, depending on the location of the pleural effusion. Normal breath sounds are heard on the contralateral side over healthy lung tissue. The diminished breath sounds have a low pitch that can be heard using either the bell or diaphragm of the stethoscope.

7. Premature dynamic compression of the large central airways and the loss of elastic tension in the lung tissue limit airflow during expiration. Increased intrinsic airway resistance may also be present. Increased amounts of air trapped in the lungs change the acoustical qualities of the sound transmitted, creating a mismatch between the pleurae and chest wall, and the hyperinflated lung tissue. Consequently, breath sounds are diminished.

8. Diminished or absent breath sounds associated with chronic obstructive pulmonary disease are heard over the anterior, posterior, and lateral chest wall surfaces. If the breath sounds are audible, they're soft in intensity and have a low pitch that's heard best using the diaphragm of the stethoscope. The sounds are heard throughout inspiration and expiration.

9. Breath sounds are normally attenuated and filtered at the pleural surface. In an obese person, a thickened chest wall increases the distance between lung tissue and the chest wall surface. This results in additional filtering of the breath sounds as they are transmitted from the pleurae to the chest wall surface.

10. Adding positive end-expiratory pressure (PEEP) during mechanical ventilation of an intubated patient can diminish breath sounds in the following way: PEEP increases functional residual capacity (FRC), the amount of air remaining in the airways at the end of normal expiration. Increasing FRC hyperinflates the lungs. Increased amounts of air in the small airways and alveoli change the acoustical qualities of the sound transmitted through the chest wall, creating a mismatch between the pleurae and chest wall, and the hyperinflated lung.

18 Classifying adventitious sounds

1. Coarse crackles are discontinuous, explosive sounds that are loud and low-pitched.

2. Fine crackles are discontinuous, explosive sounds that are shorter in duration, higher in pitch, and less intense than coarse crackles.

3. Wheezes are continuous sounds that are high-pitched and have a hissing or coughing sound. They commonly have a musical quality.

4. Low-pitched wheezes are continuous sounds that are low-pitched and commonly resemble snoring.

19 Adventitious sounds: Crackles

1. The timing of crackles is described as early inspiration, midinspiration, or late inspiration or early expiration, midexpiration, or late expiration. Pitch is usually described as high or low. Intensity varies and is described as loud or soft. Density is described as profuse or scanty. The duration, indicating the length of time that the crackles can be heard during inspiration or expiration, varies.

2. The conditions associated with late inspiratory crackles include atelectasis, resolving lobar pneumonia, interstitial fibrosis, and left-sided heart failure.

3. The crackles associated with atelectasis begin late in inspiration and become more profuse toward the end of inspiration. They vary in intensity but are high-pitched. Because crackles associated with atelectasis are poorly transmitted to the chest wall surface, their intensity and density change when the stethoscope is moved only a short distance. They aren't audible at the mouth. The patient's position also affects these crackles. For example, in an immobile patient, profuse crackles are heard in the dependent lung regions, but crackles are absent or scanty in the nondependent lung regions. Also, crackles associated with atelectasis may clear somewhat with coughing.

4. Crackles associated with lobar pneumonia begin late in inspiration and become more profuse toward the end of inspiration. These crackles are typically high-pitched.

5. Diffuse interstitial fibrosis impairs or destroys alveoli by filling them with abnormal cells or by scarring the lung tissue. Unaffected alveoli are usually hyperaerated. The lungs become stiff and more difficult to inflate, and airflow volumes usually decrease. Theoretically, the delayed opening of small airways during inspiration causes alveolar pressures in the affected lung tissue to fall more significantly than in healthy alveoli. This fall in alveolar pressures leads to an increased pressure gradient that generates repetitive late inspiratory crackles.

6. Left-sided heart failure leads to fluid accumulation in the lung interstitium. Crackles are produced by the rapid equalization of pressures associated with the delayed opening of airways narrowed by pulmonary edema.

7. Coarse crackles are thought to be produced by the intermittent closure of large bronchi and the corresponding flow of a bolus of air through the obstructed area.

8. Early inspiratory crackles are associated with excessive mucus production in patients with chronic bronchitis. The proliferation and hypertrophy of mucous glands within the airways are caused by chronic exposure to airway irritants, such as cigarette smoke and air pollution.

9. In patients with bronchiectasis, crackles tend to be profuse, low-pitched, heard during early inspiration or midinspiration, and coarser than those associated with chronic bronchitis. Coughing may decrease the number of crackles heard, but position changes don't affect them.

10. Pleural crackles are heard on the chest wall over the affected area. Their intensity is loud, and they have a coarse, grating quality and a low pitch. Their duration is discontinuous. They may be heard during inspiration only or during both the inspiratory and expiratory phases of the respiratory cycle.

20 Adventitious sounds: Wheezes

1. Wheezes are musical sounds generated by air passing through a bronchus so narrowed as to be almost closed. The bronchus walls oscillate between closed and barely open positions; these oscillations generate audible sounds.

2. Wheezes are high-pitched, continuous sounds with frequencies of 200 Hz or greater and a duration of 250 ms or more. Their duration is long enough to carry an audible pitch similar to a musical tone. Wheezes are described by their timing within the respiratory cycle: They may be heard during inspiration or expiration or continuously throughout the respiratory cycle. They can be further described as localized or diffuse, episodic or chronic.

3. The conditions associated with wheezes include bronchospasm, airway thickening caused by mucosal swelling or muscle hypertrophy, inhalation of a foreign object, tumor, secretions, or dynamic airway compression.

4. Expiratory polyphonic wheezes are usually heard over the anterior, posterior, and lateral chest wall surfaces during expiration. Their intensity is usually described as loud and musical, and their duration is continuous. They have a high pitch that's heard best using the diaphragm of the stethoscope.

5. Fixed monophonic wheezes, which have a constant pitch and a single musical tone, are generated by the oscillations of a large, partially obstructed bronchus. The obstruction may be caused by a tumor, a foreign body, bronchial stenosis, or an intrabronchial granuloma.

6. Sequential inspiratory wheezes are sometimes heard over the lung bases in patients with interstitial fibrosis, asbestosis, or fibrosing alveolitis.

7. The monophonic wheezes are generated by airways that open late in inspiration in unaerated lung regions. The rapid inflow of air precipitates airway wall vibrations, generating sequential inspiratory wheezes.

8. Airways narrowed by bronchospasm or mucosal swelling produce single or multiple monophonic wheezes that may occur during inspiration or expiration or throughout the respiratory cycle.

9. The progressive airway obstruction that occurs in patients with status asthmaticus can cause a dynamic pattern of wheezing. First, monophonic wheezes are heard only during expiration; then they are heard throughout the respiratory cycle. As status asthmaticus becomes more severe, all wheezes heard over the chest wall surfaces disappear because a combination of air trapping and severe airway narrowing causes the site of dynamic airway compression to move toward the lung periphery. This phenomenon is called a silent chest.

10. Stridor is a loud musical sound that's heard at a distance from the patient, usually without a stethoscope.

Selected readings

Anatomy & Physiology Made Incredibly Easy, 4th ed. Philadelphia: Lippincott Williams & Wilkins, 2010.

Assessment Made Incredibly Easy, 5th ed. Philadelphia: Lippincott Williams & Wilkins, 2013.

Bickley, L.S., and Szilagyi, P.G. *Bates Guide to Physical Examination and History Taking*, 10th ed. Philadelphia: Lippincott Williams & Wilkins, 2009.

Chattterjee, K. (2012a). Auscultation of cardiac murmurs. In: *UpToDate,* Otto, C.M. (ed.). Retrieved from www.uptodate.com.

Chatterjee, K. (2012b). Auscultation of heart sounds. In: *UpToDate,* Otto, C.M. (ed.). Retrieved from www.uptodate.com

Cottrell, D. "Action Stat: Iatrogenic Pneumothorax." *Nursing* 40(3):72, 2010.

Daines, J.E., et al. *Advanced Health Assessment and Clinical Diagnosis in Primary Care*, 4th ed. St. Louis: Mosby, 2012.

Ferns, T., and West, S. "The Art of Auscultation: Evaluating a Patient's Respiratory Pathology." *British Journal of Nursing* 17(12):772–777, 2008.

Holditch-Davis, D. et al. "Predictors of Wheezing in Prematurely Born Children." *Journal of Obstetric, Gynecologic, and Neonatal Nursing* 37(7):262–273, 2008.

http://www.littmann.com/wps/portal/3M/ en_US/3M-Littmann/stethoscope/ littmann-learning-institute/heart-lung-sounds/ accessed 1/12/2013

Kritek, P., and Choi, A. Approach to the patient with disease of the respiratory system. In: Long, D.L., Fauci, A.S., Kasper, D.L., Hauser, S.L., Jameson, J.L.,

Loscalzo, J., eds. *Harrison's Principles of Internal Medicine.* 18th ed. New York: McGraw-Hill, 2012.

Light, R.W. (2012, May). Pneumothorax. In: *The Merck Manual.* Retrieved from http:// www.merckmanuals.com/professional/ pulmonary_disorders/mediastinal_and_ pleural_disorders/pneumothorax.html

Mangla, A. (2012). *Heart sounds.* Retrieved on January 14, 2013, from http://emedicine.medscape.com/ article/1894036-overview.

McCool, F.D., and Tzelepis, G.E. "Dysfunction of the Diaphragm." *New England Journal of Medicine* 366:932–942, 2012. DOI: 10.1056/NEJMra1007236

Midozi, W.K., et al. "Predictors for Wheezing Phenotypes in the First Decade of Life." *Respirology* 13(4):537–545, 2008.

Morrison, B., Nickerson, M., and Pollard, M. "Simulation in Nursing Staff Development: A Concept Analysis." *Journal of Nurses in Staff Development* 27(2):81–89, 2011.

Nishimura, R.A., et al. "ACC/AHA 2008 Guideline Update on Valvular Heart Disease: Focused Update on Infective Endocarditis." *Journal of American College of Cardiology* 52(8):676–685, 2008.

Stahlheber, C.L., and Mosenifar, Z. (2012). *Breath sound assessment.* Retrieved from http://emedicine.medscape.com/ article/1894146

Wagner, C. (2012). *Advanced respiratory assessment in the school-aged child.* Retrieved from www.childrens.com advanced-respiratory-assessment-school-aged-...

Additional web site

www.rch.org.au/kidsinfo/fact_sheets/Voice_disorders
(Accessed February 1, 2013).

Glossary

A₂ *abbr* Aortic component of S_2.

Accessory muscles of respiration
Muscles involved in labored, or forceful, breathing. They include the sternocleidomastoid, scalene, trapezius, rhomboid, and abdominal muscles.

Acoustical mismatch Phenomenon in which sounds transmitted through two different media, such as air and tissue, are diminished in intensity or blocked.

Acute pulmonary hypertension Sudden increased pressure within the pulmonary circulation (above 30 mm Hg systolic and 12 mm Hg diastolic).

Adult respiratory distress syndrome (ARDS) Disease with numerous causes that's characterized by interstitial and alveolar edema and progressive hypoxemia; also known as *shock lung* or *posttraumatic lung*.

Adventitious sound An acquired (usually) abnormal sound superimposed over normal breath sounds.

AES *abbr* Aortic ejection sound.

Alveolar-capillary membrane Cell membrane across which oxygen and carbon dioxide must diffuse for respiration to occur.

Alveolar duct The narrowed end portion of the bronchioles that terminate in clusters of alveolar sacs.

Alveolus One of the millions of small, saclike lung structures where oxygen–carbon dioxide exchange occurs.

Amplitude Magnitude or intensity of a sound or pulsation.

Anatomic dead space Air that remains in the conducting airways during each breath. This air isn't involved in oxygen–carbon dioxide exchange.

Antigen Substance or material foreign to the body that causes a reaction leading to the formation of antibodies.

Aortic ejection sound Opening sound of a stenotic aortic valve. It follows S_1 early in ventricular systole and appears just after the QRS complex on the ECG.

Aortic regurgitation Abnormal condition of turbulent backward blood flow through the aortic valve into the left ventricle during diastole.

Aortic stenosis Narrowing or constriction of the aortic valve or of the aorta itself.

Aortic valve Membranous folds that prevent blood reflux from the aorta into the left ventricle.

Aortic valvular stenosis Constriction of or damage to the aortic valve that restricts forward blood flow from the left ventricle to the aorta during systole.

ARDS *abbr* Acute respiratory distress syndrome.

Arteriovenous shunt Direct passage of blood from arteries to veins, bypassing the capillary bed. This can refer to a physiologic response of the body or to an abnormal condition sometimes caused by trauma or surgery.

Asbestosis Lung disease characterized by pulmonary inflammation and fibrosis; caused by prolonged asbestos exposure.

Ascending aortic aneurysm Dilation of the thoracic portion of the aorta.

Aspiration Breathing in of foreign materials.

Asthma Disease characterized by bronchial inflammation, bronchospasm, and bronchial hyperactivity, which lead to obstructed airflow, wheezing, and shortness of breath.

Atelectasis Incomplete expansion of the lung tissue, usually caused by pressure from exudate, fluid, tumor, or an obstructed airway; may involve a lung segment or an entire lobe.

Atrial septal defect Imperfection, failure to develop fully, or absence of the dividing wall (septum) between the heart's atria.

Atrioventricular node Small mass of specialized cardiac tissue, located in the lower portion of the right atrium near the septum, that transmits electrical impulses from the sinoatrial node to the bundle of His.

Atrioventricular valves Valves between the atria and the ventricles—specifically, the tricuspid valve of the heart's right side and the mitral valve of the heart's left side.

Attenuation Decrease in the intensity or loudness of a breath sound.

Auscultation Act of listening to sounds made by the body; usually performed with a stethoscope.

Austin Flint murmur Diastolic heart sound generated by turbulent blood flow across the mitral valve; caused by aortic regurgitation, which closes the mitral leaflets.

AV *abbr* Atrioventricular.

Axillary fold One of the two anatomic landmarks anterior and posterior to the armpit, formed by the normal contour of the skin over the pectoralis major muscle anteriorly and the latissimus dorsi muscle posteriorly.

Ball-in-cage valve Prosthetic heart valve characterized by a caged ball that moves with ventricular pressure to open and close a valvular opening.

Bell Cup-shaped portion of the stethoscope that's best suited for listening to low-pitched sounds.

Bifurcate To divide into two branches.

Bileaflet valve (1) Prosthetic heart valve characterized by two small wings that control blood flow; (2) mitral valve.

Binaural headpiece Stethoscope headpiece that supplies sounds to both ears simultaneously.

Blowing Term used to describe a continuous murmur sound, like the sound of air passing through pursed lips.

Booming Term used to describe a deep, resonant heart sound that's sudden and percussive.

Bronchial circulation Oxygenated blood that arises from the aorta or subclavicular artery and supplies the tracheobronchial tree with oxygen and nutrients.

Bronchial gland One of the glands secreting mucus and serous liquid in the tracheobronchial tree. These glands are most numerous in the medium-sized bronchi and are the main source of bronchial secretions.

Bronchiectasis Irreversible dilation of the bronchi characterized by chronic cough, sputum production, fibrosis, and atelectatic lung tissue surrounding the affected airways.

Bronchophony Voice sound with increased tone or clarity in vocal resonance auscultated over the chest wall.

Bronchospasm Smooth muscle contraction within the airway walls, which leads to airway narrowing and reduced airflow and may be accompanied by coughing and wheezing.

Bronchovesicular breath sound Normal breath sound auscultated between the mainstem bronchi and lung periphery; also known as a *transitional breath sound*.

Bundle of His Small band of specialized cardiac muscle fibers located in the intraventricular septum that relay the atrial electrical impulses to the ventricles.

Capillary hydrostatic pressure Fluid pressure within the capillary system, which, when elevated, leads to fluid extravasation out of the capillary system into the interstitium.

Cardiac cycle Sequence of events (systole and diastole) that enables the heart to receive and pump blood.

Cardiac output Quantity of oxygenated blood pumped through the body by the heart, usually expressed in liters per minute. Is computed as stroke volume × heart rate.

Cardiac tamponade Heart compression caused by effusion or collection of fluid in the pericardium, resulting in decreased cardiac output.

Cervical venous hum murmur Murmur caused by rapid downward blood flow through the jugular veins in the lower part of the neck.

Chordae tendineae Tendinous cords that connect each cusp of the two atrioventricular valves to appropriate papillary muscles in the ventricles.

Chronic bronchitis Disease characterized by chronic cough and sputum production that persists for at least 3 months and occurs 2 years in a row.

Chronic obstructive pulmonary disease (COPD) Chronic lung disease characterized by obstructed bronchial airflow or exhalation. Chronic bronchitis, emphysema, and asthma are types of obstructive lung disease.

Cilia Motile, whiplike extensions from cell surfaces. Ciliated columnar epithelial cells line the walls of the tracheobronchial tree.

Click Short heart sound; also, another term for a midsystolic sound that occurs when a prolapsed mitral valve's leaflet and chordae tendineae tense.

Click-murmur syndrome Condition in which a click is followed by a murmur, as in mitral valve prolapse syndrome.

Closing click Heart sound generated by valve closure. Closing clicks are heard with all prosthetic valves, regardless of their type or position.

Coarctation of the aorta Localized aortic malformation characterized by deformity of the aortic media and causing severe narrowing of the aortic lumen.

Compliance Tissue's or organ's ability to yield to pressure without disruption; commonly used to describe the distensibility of an air- or fluid-filled organ, such as the heart or lungs.

Conchae Shell-shaped turbinate bones in the nasal cavity that stimulate turbulent airflow within the nasal passages. The dense mucus and capillary beds that line the turbinates' surface encourage warming and humidification of inspired air.

Conducting airway One of the airways beginning at the nose and ending at the terminal bronchioles. These airways are responsible for transporting air during breathing but are not involved in oxygen–carbon dioxide exchange.

Conduction system Specialized cardiac cells and fibers that initiate and/or relay the electrical impulses, stimulating the heart muscle to contract.

Configuration Shape of a murmur's sound as recorded on a phonocardiogram; one of the characteristics used to describe murmurs.

Congestion Abnormal accumulation of fluid or blood in an organ or organ part.

Consolidation Inflammatory solidification of lung tissue.

Constrictive pericarditis Inflammation of the pericardium that leads to thickening and possible calcification of the pericardial sac, resulting in impaired diastolic filling, inflow stasis, or a constrictive effect.

Continuous murmur Murmur that begins in systole and persists, without interruption, through S_2 into diastole.

Contractile cell One of the myocardial cells that contract to start systole. These cells depolarize and repolarize by means of ion flow.

Contralateral Referring to the opposite side or opposing symmetrical structure.

COPD *abbr* Chronic obstructive pulmonary disease.

Cor pulmonale Heart disease caused by pulmonary hypertension secondary to disease of the lung or its blood vessels, resulting in hypertrophy of the right ventricle.

Crackles Adventitious lung sounds characterized by a short, explosive or popping sound usually heard during inspiration; described as *coarse* (loud and low in pitch) or *fine* (less intense and high in pitch); formerly known as a *rale*.

Crepitation Crackling sound that resembles the sound made by rubbing hair between two fingers.

Crescendo Term used to describe the configuration of a murmur that increases in intensity.

Crescendo–decrescendo Term used to describe the configuration of a murmur that rises in intensity and then fades away.

Cusp One of the triangular segments of a cardiac valve or one of the semilunar segments of the aortic or pulmonary valve.

Dampened Diminished sound intensity or amplitude; term used to describe sounds.

Decrescendo Term used to describe the configuration of a murmur that decreases in intensity.

Dependent lung regions Lowest lung regions (the lung bases when the patient is upright).

Depolarization Movement of sodium ions into a contractile cell, creating a positive charge inside the cell.

Diamond-shaped murmur Crescendo–decrescendo murmur.

Diaphragm Primary muscle of respiration, which separates the thoracic and abdominal cavities; also the part of the stethoscope used to auscultate for high-pitched sounds.

Diastole Expansion of the ventricles occurring in the interval between S_2 and S_1. The heart muscle, relaxing, fills with blood during this part of the cardiac cycle.

Diffuse Widely distributed; not localized.

Dilation of pulmonic valve ring Expansion of a valve aperture. A dilated pulmonic valve can contribute to a Graham Steell murmur.

Distribution of ventilation Movement or circulation of air to specific lung regions during breathing.

Dull percussion note Deadened, or nonresonant, sound heard when a solid organ or dense body part is percussed.

Duration Length of time a heart or breath sound is heard; one of the six characteristics used to describe heart sounds.

Dynamic airway compression Narrowing of the airways during expiration caused by properties of intrapleural pressure, radial traction exerted by lung parenchyma, and the loss of elastic recoil within the lung.

Dynamic obstruction Blocked outflow from one of the heart's chambers that can be demonstrated only during myocardial contraction or systole.

Dyspnea Difficult or labored breathing.

Early diastolic aortic regurgitation Blood backflow from the aorta that occurs early in diastole, when the ventricle is resting and filling with oxygenated blood.

ECG *abbr* Electrocardiogram; also written as EKG.

Ectopic beats Arrhythmic heartbeats arising from places other than the heart's normal pacemaker, the sinoatrial node.

Edema Excessive accumulation of fluid in intercellular tissue spaces of the body.

Egophony Voice sound that has a nasal or bleating quality when auscultated over the chest wall; "ee" is heard as "ay"; an "A" to "E" change.

Ejection sound Sound caused by the opening of a stenotic aortic or pulmonic valve, usually occurring early in systole.

Ejection velocity Measure of the speed of blood flow.

Elastic recoil Spontaneous contraction of lung parenchyma that occurs during expiration and that helps move air out of the lungs.

Elastic tension Support and traction exerted on the airways because of the natural elastic recoil properties of the surrounding lung parenchyma.

Epicardial pacing Regulation of the rate of heart muscle contraction by an artificial cardiac pacemaker stimulating the heart through electrical leads attached to the heart surface.

Epiglottis Small elastic cartilage attached at the larynx that covers the opening to the trachea during swallowing.

Equal pressure point Point in the airways where intrapulmonary and intrapleural pressures are equal.

ES *abbr* Ejection sound.

Exudate Inflammatory fluid leaked from body cells or tissues.

Fibrosis Abnormal formation of fibrous connective tissue that usually occurs as a reparative or reactive process within an organ or tissue but ultimately replaces healthy, functional tissue.

5LMCL *abbr* Fifth intercostal space, left midclavicular line (mitral area).

5LSB *abbr* Fifth intercostal space, left sternal border (tricuspid area).

FRC *abbr* Functional residual capacity.

Frequency Pitch of a breath sound measured in hertz.

Functional murmur Benign murmur that doesn't impair heart function.

Gallop rhythm Triple rhythms; the S_1, S_2, S_3 sequence; the S_4, S_1, S_2 sequence; or both. Sounds like a horse's gallop.

Gas exchange surface Alveolar capillary surface that's actively involved in diffusing oxygen and carbon dioxide.

Graham Steell murmur Pulmonic regurgitation murmur caused by pulmonic hypertension and pulmonic valve ring dilation.

Heart failure Clinical syndrome caused by left-sided or right-sided heart dysfunction. Left-sided heart failure results in pulmonary edema and breathlessness. Right-sided heart failure results in liver congestion, increased venous pressure, and peripheral edema.

Hemidiaphragm One-half of the diaphragm (either the right or left side).

High-output condition Physiologic state that causes or results in increased cardiac output.

Hila Medial lung aspects where the bronchi, nerves, and vessels enter and leave.

Holodiastolic Pertaining to the entire diastole; used to describe a murmur that persists throughout diastole.

Holosystolic Pertaining to the entire systole; used to describe a murmur that persists throughout systole; also known as *pansystolic*.

Holosystolic mitral regurgitation Blood backflow that's caused by an incompetent mitral valve and that can be heard throughout systole.

Hyperinflation Overinflation of the lung that occurs with air trapping in obstructive lung diseases, such as emphysema.

Hypertrophic cardiomyopathy Narrowing or constriction of the left ventricle's subaortic region caused by tissue enlargement in that area; also known as *idiopathic hypertrophic subaortic stenosis*. This condition can be a cause of subvalvular aortic stenosis.

Hypertrophy Enlargement or overgrowth of an entire organ or of part of an organ, caused by an increase in the size of its constituent cells.

Hypoxemia Abnormally low oxygen tension in arterial blood.

Hz *abbr* Hertz.

Idiopathic Of unknown cause.

I:E ratio *abbr* Inspiratory–expiratory ratio.

Impedance matching Similar acoustical characteristics of two organs or types of tissue that allow effective sound transmission.

Incompetent valve Heart valve that cannot perform its functions because of congenital defects, disease, or trauma.

Infective endocarditis Inflammation of the endocardium caused by infection with microorganisms (bacteria or fungi); primarily affects the heart valves.

Inferior vena cava Venous trunk for the lower extremities and the pelvic and abdominal viscera.

Inspiratory–expiratory ratio Numerical expression of the duration of inspiration in relation to the duration of expiration.

Intensity Degree of loudness; one of the six characteristics used to describe heart sounds.

Intercostal muscle Muscle found between the ribs. Internal and external intercostal muscles help stabilize and expand or lower the rib cage with ventilation.

Internodal pathway One of the fibers connecting the small masses of tissue that transmit the electrical impulses setting the heart's rate and rhythm.

Interstitial fibrosis Abnormal formation of fibrous tissue that occurs as a reparative or reactive process within the alveolar septa and interstitial areas of the lungs.

Interstitium Small gap in an organ or a tissue; in lung parenchyma, the space between the alveolar and capillary membranes.

Interventricular septum Dividing wall between the heart's ventricles.

Intrapleural pressure Relative pressure that occurs between the pleurae. Negative pressure occurs during inspiration; positive pressure occurs during expiration.

Intrapulmonary pressure Pressure within the lung. Negative pressure causes air to flow inward; positive pressure causes air to move outward.

Isovolumic contraction Initial period in early systole when the atrioventricular and semilunar valves are closed and intraventricular pressures rise but blood has not yet been ejected from the ventricles.

Isovolumic relaxation Brief period in early diastole when the atrioventricular and semilunar valves are closed, just before the atrioventricular valves open and passive filling of the ventricles begins.

Laminar airflow Orderly, linear airflow.

Larynx Cartilaginous organ located between the pharynx and the trachea that houses the vocal cords and allows for voice production.

LBBB *abbr* Left bundle branch block.

Leaflet Structure resembling a small leaf, especially a heart valve's cusps.

Left atrial shunt Small amount of deoxygenated blood that returns to the left atrium; normally, this is venous return from bronchial circulation.

Left bundle branch block Interrupted conduction through the fiber that activates the left ventricle, resulting in a prolonged or abnormal QRS complex.

Left lateral recumbent position Position that brings the heart's apex closer to the chest wall for auscultation. The patient lies on his left side, with his right knee and thigh drawn up to his chest.

Left mainstem bronchus One of the two main branches extending from the trachea that supplies air to the left lung. It leaves the trachea at a sharper angle than the right mainstem bronchus and passes under the aortic arch before entering the lung.

Left-sided heart failure Inability of the left ventricle to pump blood adequately, causing decreased cardiac output, which results in pulmonary congestion and edema.

Left ventricular decompensation Failure of the left ventricle's myocardium to contract and maintain adequate cardiac output.

Left ventricular hypertrophy Enlargement of the left ventricle's myocardium, which can result in reduced or abnormal ventricular functioning.

Left ventricular outflow obstruction Stenosis or other blockage preventing flow of oxygenated blood from the left ventricle into the aorta.

Left ventricular pressure overload Increased pressure within the left ventricle that impairs its ability to function normally; commonly caused by excessively elevated systemic blood pressure.

Left ventricular volume overload Excessive volume within the left ventricle that causes it to become distended and impairs its ability to function normally.

Lobar Referring to or involving any lung lobe.

Location Site at which a breath or a heart sound can be auscultated.

Lower airway *See* Tracheobronchial tree.

Low-pitched wheeze Continuous, low-pitched sound that resembles snoring; previously classified as a sonorous bronchus or a sonorous rale.

M$_1$ *abbr* Mitral component of S$_1$.

Macrophage Large ameboid, mononuclear cell that acts as a defense mechanism against infection; one of the three cell types lining the alveoli.

Mainstem bronchi breath sound Harsh, tubular (hollow) breath sound heard over a mainstem bronchus; also known as *rhonchi*.

Mast cell Connective tissue cell whose specific physiologic function remains unknown. The secretory mast cells on the surface of the large airways may be stimulated or affected by drugs, hormones, antigens, or other messenger cells to precipitate or control bronchoconstriction.

Mean airflow velocity Air flow rates occurring within an airway during the middle part of exhalation.

Mechanical ventilation Breathing that's assisted or controlled by a machine (a ventilator).

Mediastinal crunch Heart sound created by heart movement against air in the mediastinum; also known as *Hamman sign*.

Mediastinum Tissues separating the two lungs, between the sternum and the vertebral column and from the thoracic inlet to the diaphragm. It contains the heart and its vessels, the trachea, esophagus, thymus, lymph nodes, and other organs and tissues.

Middiastolic aortic regurgitation Turbulent backward blood flow through the aorta into the left ventricle occurring midway between S_2 and S_1.

Middiastolic click Click heard midway between S_2 and S_1 in the cardiac cycle; usually associated with a stenotic or rigid atrioventricular valve.

Midsystolic ejection murmur Crisp, high-frequency sound resulting from a stenotic aortic or pulmonic valve opening in systole.

Mitral regurgitation Turbulent backward blood flow from the left ventricle into the left atrium caused by the mitral valve's inability to close completely.

Mitral stenosis Mitral valve narrowing or constriction obstructing flow of blood from the left atrium to the left ventricle.

Mitral valve Tissue folds that, when closed, prevent blood flow from the left ventricle to the left atrium; also called the *bicuspid valve*.

Mitral valve prolapse Mitral valve bulging from the proper position back toward the left atrium during systole. It can result in mitral regurgitation and may produce a late systolic murmur, possibly with a nonejection midsystolic click.

Monophonic Having one distinct musical sound or tone; used to describe selected wheezes.

MSC *abbr* Midsystolic click.

Mucus Serous, watery liquid secreted by bronchial glands and goblet cells within the airways.

Murmur Sound heard during auscultation that results from vibrations produced by blood moving within the heart and adjacent blood vessels; may be benign or abnormal.

Myocardial infarction Tissue death in the heart's muscle; usually caused by inadequate coronary artery perfusion.

Myocardium Heart wall, comprising cardiac muscle tissue.

Nonejection click Click caused by a valve that isn't associated with movement of blood through or across the valve; commonly used to describe the click of mitral valve prolapse.

Normal breath sound Sound auscultated over chest wall areas of a healthy person.

Normal sinus rhythm Normal physiologic heart rhythm originating in the sinoatrial node; usually considered to be 60 to 100 beats/minute.

O_2–CO_2 exchange *abbr* Oxygen–carbon dioxide exchange.

Opening click Opening sound created by some prosthetic heart valves or by a diseased valve.

Opening snap Sound created by mitral valve leaflets that have become stenotic or abnormally narrowed but that are still somewhat mobile.

OS *abbr* Opening snap.

Oscillation Vibration, fluctuation.

P_2 *abbr* Pulmonic component of S_2.

Papillary muscle Muscular protrusion, or projection, in the ventricles that attaches to and regulates the atrioventricular valves by way of the chordae tendineae.

Parasympathetic nervous system Part of the involuntary nervous system that supplies innervation to the internal organs.

The hormone mediator is acetylcholine. The vagus nerve is a parasympathetic nerve that innervates the airways and, when stimulated, causes smooth muscle contraction, cough, and mucus discharge from the bronchial glands.

Parenchyma Functioning cells of an organ that distinguish or determine the primary organ function.

Patent ductus arteriosus Abnormal channel connecting the pulmonary artery to the descending aorta; results in arterial blood recirculation through the lungs.

PCG *abbr* Phonocardiogram.

PDA *abbr* Patent ductus arteriosus.

PEEP *abbr* Positive end-expiratory pressure.

Perfusion Blood flow to or through an organ or tissue supplied by the blood vessels.

Pericardial fluid Fluid in the space between the visceral and parietal layers of the pericardium.

Pericardial friction rub Characteristic high-pitched friction noise created by inflamed or dry pericardial surfaces rubbing together.

Pericardial knock S_3 associated with constrictive pericarditis.

Pericarditis Inflammation of the pericardium.

Pericardium Two-layer fibrous sac that surrounds the heart and the roots of the great vessels consisting of the visceral and parietal layers.

Peripheral Toward the outer boundary or perimeter; not central.

Peripheral vascular resistance Resistance to the passage of blood through the small blood vessels, especially the arterioles, caused by friction between the blood and the blood vessel wall.

Pharynx Musculomembranous passage between the posterior nares and the larynx and esophagus; also referred to as the *throat*. It serves as a joint conduit for food and air.

Phonation Production of vocal sounds.

Phonocardiogram Graphic record of heart sounds and murmurs, including pulse tracings, produced by phonocardiography.

Physiologic S_3 S_3 that isn't associated with an abnormal condition; often found in young individuals.

Pitch A tone's vibration or frequency, measured in cycles per second as sound amplitude; subjectively described as high, medium, or low.

Plateau-shaped murmur Murmur in which intensity is the same, or flat, throughout its duration.

Pleurae Thin, serous membranes that surround the lungs (visceral pleura) and line the thoracic cavity's inner walls (parietal pleura).

Pleural crackle Loud, grating sound caused by inflamed or damaged pleurae; also called *pleural friction rub*.

Pleural effusion Abnormal accumulation of fluid between visceral and parietal pleurae.

Pleural friction rub Sound created by friction between the parietal and visceral pleurae surrounding the lungs; similar to a pericardial friction rub.

PMI *abbr* Point of maximum impulse.

Pneumonia Inflammation of the lung parenchyma.

Pneumothorax Accumulation of air within the pleural cavity.

Point of maximum impulse Chest wall site where the heartbeat can be seen or felt most strongly; typically located over the heart's apex.

Polyphonic Having multiple distinct musical sounds or tones; used to describe selected wheezes.

Porcine valve Prosthetic heart valve made from swine (pig) products.

Positive end-expiratory pressure Application of positive pressure to exhalation during mechanical ventilation; used to help prevent expiratory airway collapse and thus improve oxygenation.

Pressure gradient Difference in pressure between two regions.

P-R interval Time between atrial depolarization and ventricular depolarization, as recorded on the ECG. The P-R interval begins at the onset of the P wave and lasts until the onset of the QRS complex. Ordinarily, atrial contraction occurs during the P-R interval.

Prosthetic valve Artificial heart valve replacing a nonfunctional valve. Ball-in-cage, bileaflet, porcine, and tilting-disk are the four kinds of prosthetic heart valves.

Pulmonary artery Blood vessel leading from the right ventricle to the lungs.

Pulmonary artery dilation Expansion or stretching of the pulmonary artery beyond its normal dimensions.

Pulmonary circulation Blood pumped by the right ventricle into the pulmonary artery that circulates through the pulmonary capillary beds, where gas exchange occurs. The oxygenated blood is carried to the left atrium via the pulmonary veins.

Pulmonary edema Excessive accumulation of fluid within the lung.

Pulmonary hypertension Increased blood pressure within the pulmonary circulatory system.

Pulmonary vein One of the four veins that return oxygenated blood from the lungs to the heart's left atrium.

Pulmonic ejection sound High-pitched click commonly created by the opening of a stenotic pulmonic valve. It is the only right-sided heart sound whose intensity increases during expiration and decreases during inspiration.

Pulmonic regurgitation Abnormal condition of backward blood flow across the pulmonic valve during diastole.

Pulmonic stenosis Narrowing or constriction of the pulmonic valve or the region just above or below the valve.

Pulmonic valvular stenosis Narrowing or constriction of the pulmonic valve.

Purkinje fibers Modified cardiac muscle cells found beneath the endocardium. They are part of the heart's electrical impulse–conducting system.

P wave Part of the ECG tracing that represents atrial depolarization.

QRS complex ECG waves representing the spread of electrical impulses from the

bundle branches to the ventricular muscle. The QRS complex corresponds to ventricular depolarization.

Quality Heart sound characteristic determined by a combination of the sound's frequencies; one of the six characteristics used to describe heart sounds. A sound's quality may be described as sharp, dull, booming, snapping, blowing, harsh, or musical.

Radiation Spread of a heart sound beyond its area of origin.

Rales *See* Crackles.

RBBB *abbr* Right bundle branch block.

Regurgitant murmur Sound created by turbulent backward blood flow through an incompetent heart valve.

Repolarization Movement of calcium ions into the cell and potassium ions out of the cell, followed by the extrusion of sodium and calcium ions from the cell and the restoration of potassium ions into the cell by the sodium–potassium pump.

Resistance Force that hinders motion; hindrance or impedance.

Resonance Sound quality produced by percussing structures or cavities that radiate sound vibrations and energy.

Respiratory cycle One complete cycle of inspiration and expiration.

Rheumatic heart disease Valvular abnormalities that are an aftereffect of rheumatic fever; most commonly, mitral, tricuspid, or aortic stenosis and insufficiency.

Rhonchus *See* Low-pitched wheeze; plural form: Rhonchi.

Right bundle branch block Interrupted conduction through the fiber that activates the right ventricle, resulting in a prolonged QRS complex.

Right mainstem bronchus One of the two main branches extending from the trachea that supplies air to the right lung. It leaves the trachea at a less-acute angle than the left mainstem bronchus and is a more likely landing site for aspirated foreign bodies.

Right-sided heart failure Inability of the right ventricle to function properly.

Right-sided S$_3$ Heart sound caused by a noncompliant right ventricle and high right atrial pressure. It's heard in patients with cor pulmonale, pulmonary embolism, right-sided heart failure secondary to mitral stenosis with left-sided heart failure or pulmonary hypertension, and severe tricuspid insufficiency.

Right-sided S$_4$ S$_4$ generated in the right ventricle; commonly heard with conditions that create pressures greater than 100mm Hg in that ventricle. It may accompany such conditions as pulmonic stenosis, pulmonary hypertension, or sudden tricuspid regurgitation.

Right ventricular outflow obstruction Stenosis, embolus, or other blockage preventing flow of deoxygenated blood from the right ventricle into the pulmonary artery.

S$_1$ *abbr* First heart sound; produced by closure of the mitral (M$_1$) and tricuspid (T$_1$) valves.

S$_2$ *abbr* Second heart sound; produced by closure of the aortic (A$_2$) and pulmonic (P$_2$) valves.

S$_3$ *abbr* Third heart sound; created by vibrations caused by the rapid, passive filling of the ventricles. S$_3$ is abnormal in adults older than age 20. The cadence is similar to the word *Tennessee*.

S$_4$ *abbr* Fourth heart sound; generated by stretching and filling of a ventricle during late diastole; associated with atrial contraction. The cadence is similar to the word *Kentucky*.

SA *abbr* Sinoatrial.

Sarcoidosis Granulomatous disease of unknown origin that may cause pulmonary fibrosis.

Scapula Triangular flat bone that makes up part of the shoulder girdle; also known as the *shoulder blade*.

Segmental bronchus Airway that branches from a lobar bronchus and conducts air to a lung segment.

SEM *abbr* Systolic ejection murmur (also referred to as SM).

Semilunar valves Crescent-shaped heart valves between the ventricles and the pulmonary artery and aorta.

Serous Having a watery consistency.

Shunting Abnormal communication between the high-pressure arterial system and the low-pressure venous system.

Silent chest Absence of breath sounds during auscultation; usually associated with severe bronchospasm and insufficient airflow to produce sounds.

Sinoatrial node Small mass of tissue at the junction of the superior vena cava and the right atrium that triggers the electrical impulses that begin the cardiac cycle.

SM *abbr* Systolic murmur (also referred to as SEM).

Snap Short, sharp heart sound associated with sudden closing or opening of a heart valve.

Status asthmaticus Severe asthma that's resistant to treatment; characterized by respiratory insufficiency or failure, wheezing, and severe dyspnea.

Stenosis Narrowing or constriction of a passage, specifically a heart valve or region around the outflow tract of any of the heart's chambers.

Sternal border Auscultatory area along and to either side of the sternum.

Stethoscope Instrument used for auscultation; usually consists of a diaphragm and a bell, which are connected to one or two tubes leading to a binaural headpiece and earpieces.

Stridor Noisy, high-pitched sound that can usually be heard at a distance from the patient; caused by laryngeal spasm and mucosal swelling, which contract the vocal cords and narrow the airway.

Stroke volume Amount of blood pumped during each ventricular contraction.

Subcutaneous emphysema Presence of air or gas in the tissues beneath the skin. It results in crackling or crepitus when touched.

Subvalvular aortic stenosis murmur Murmur caused by a left ventricular outflow obstruction below the aortic valve.

Subvalvular pulmonic stenosis Narrowing or constriction of the region below the pulmonic valve.

Subvalvular pulmonic stenosis murmur
Murmur caused by a right ventricular outflow obstruction below the pulmonic valve.

Summation gallop S_4 that occurs simultaneously with S_3, thus sounding louder.

Superior vena cava Major vein that drains blood from the upper half of the body, beginning below the right costal cartilage and continuing to the right atrium.

Supine Lying on the back, face up.

Supravalvular aortic stenosis murmur Murmur caused by left ventricular outflow obstruction above the aortic valve.

Supravalvular pulmonic stenosis Narrowing or constriction of the region above the pulmonic valve.

Supravalvular pulmonic stenosis murmur Murmur caused by a right ventricular outflow obstruction above the pulmonic valve.

Surfactant Active surface agent that acts to decrease surface tension, thereby preventing alveolar collapse; believed to be secreted by type 2 alveolar cells.

Sympathetic nervous system Part of the nervous system that supplies innervation to the visceral and musculoskeletal system. Its primary hormone transmitter is norepinephrine. Sympathetic innervation to the airways facilitates smooth muscle relaxation, thereby causing bronchial dilation.

Systemic hypertension Condition in which the patient has a higher-than-normal overall blood pressure.

Systole Ventricular contraction that ejects blood into the arterial system. The left ventricle ejects into the aorta, and the right ventricle ejects into the pulmonary artery.

Systolic crescendo murmur Heart sound that begins as a faint sound and then rises in volume; occurs during the ventricular contraction phase of the cardiac cycle.

Systolic ejection murmur Murmur heard in systole that's caused by turbulent blood flow as the right or left ventricle ejects blood; it can be an innocent murmur.

Systolic regurgitation murmur Sound created by turbulent backward blood flow from either the mitral or tricuspid valve during the ventricular contraction phase of the cardiac cycle.

T_1 *abbr* Tricuspid component of S_1.

Terminal respiratory bronchioles Final part of the conducting airways. They mark the beginning of the respiratory zone.

Thoracic cavity Space within the rib cage that begins at the clavicle and ends at the diaphragm.

Thorax Bony structure that encloses the thoracic cavity, protecting the heart, lungs, and great vessels.

3LSB *abbr* Third intercostal space, left sternal border (Erb point).

Thrill Abnormal tremor felt on palpation that accompanies some vascular or cardiac murmur.

Tilting-disk valve Prosthetic heart valve characterized by a disk that tilts with ventricular pressure to open and close the valvular opening.

Tracheal breath sound Loud, tubular (hollow) breath sound auscultated over the trachea that's audible during inspiration and expiration.

Tracheobronchial tree Portion of the airway that begins at the larynx and ends at the terminal bronchioles; also known as the *lower airway*.

Tricuspid insufficiency Tricuspid valve incompetence during systole, which allows turbulent backward, or regurgitant, blood flow into the right atrium.

Tricuspid stenosis Narrowing or constriction of the tricuspid valve.

Tricuspid valve Heart valve between the right atrium and right ventricle.

Tubular breath sound Loud, hollow sound characteristically heard over the trachea and mainstem bronchi.

Turbinate *See* Conchae.

Turbulence Disturbed or irregular airflow; can be caused by rapid flow rates or variations in air pressures and velocities.

T wave Part of the ECG tracing that represents ventricular repolarization.

2LSB *abbr* Second intercostal space, left sternal border (pulmonic area).

2RSB *abbr* Second intercostal space, right sternal border (aortic area).

Type I alveolar cell One of the three cell types that make up the alveoli; covers about 95% of the alveolar surface area.

Type II alveolar cell One of the three cell types that line the alveoli; source of pulmonary surfactant.

Valsalva maneuver Attempt to exhale forcibly with the glottis closed, resulting in increased intrathoracic pressure, reduced heart rate and venous return, and increased venous pressure.

Ventilation Movement of air in and out of the lungs.

Ventricular ejection Ventricular contraction that sends blood into the arterial system; called *systole* in the cardiac cycle.

Ventricular filling Ventricular relaxation and expansion that allows blood to enter; called *diastole* in the cardiac cycle.

Ventricular outflow obstruction Blockage in the valve or vessel that carries blood out of one of the heart's ventricles.

Ventricular septal defect Opening in the septum between the ventricles; usually represents a congenital abnormality.

Ventricular tachycardia Rapid heart rate originating from one or more ectopic foci in the ventricle.

Vesicular sounds Term commonly used to describe normal breath sounds auscultated over most of the chest wall.

Vocal cord One of the two membranous structures in the larynx responsible for phonation.

Vortex Circular airflow caused by the shearing force of high-velocity airstreams alongside slower airstreams. Vortices within the airways are precipitated by airway branching that causes airflow to change direction abruptly.

Wheeze Continuous, high-pitched sound that has a musical quality; results from bronchospasm.

Whispered pectoriloquy High-frequency whispered voice sound auscultated over consolidated or atelectatic areas.

Index

i refers to an illustration; t refers to a table.

---

i refers to an illustration; t refers to a table.

---

i refers to an illustration; t refers to a table.

---

i refers to an illustration; t refers to a table.

---

i refers to an illustration; t refers to a table.